Wahlberg · Elsner · Kanerva · Maibach
Management of Positive Patch Test Reactions

Springer

Berlin
Heidelberg
New York
Hong Kong
London
Milan
Paris
Tokyo

J. E. Wahlberg · P. Elsner
L. Kanerva · H. I. Maibach
(Eds.)

Management
of Positive
Patch Test Reactions

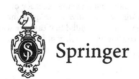 Springer

ISBN 3-540-44347-9
Springer-Verlag
Berlin
Heidelberg
New York

Library of Congress Cataloging-in-Publication Data

Management of positive patch test reactions / Jan E. Wahlberg ... [et al.].
p. cm.
Includes bibliographical references.
ISBN 3-540-44347-9 (softcover : alk. paper)
1. Contact dermatitis–Handbooks, manuals, etc. I. Wahlberg, Jan E.
RL244.M36 2003   616.97′3–dc21   2003045728

Springer-Verlag Berlin Heidelberg New York
a member of BertelsmannSpringer Science + Business Media GmbH

http://www.springer.de

© Springer-Verlag Berlin Heidelberg 2003
Printed in Germany

Cover design:
Erich Kirchner,
Heidelberg
Typesetting:
Fotosatz-Service Köhler
GmbH, Würzburg
Printing and
bookbinding:
Stürtz AG, Würzburg

Printed on acid-free paper   24/3150PF – 5 4 3 2 1 0

Preface

The International Contact Dermatitis Research
Group (ICDRG) updated their standard series
in "Proposal for a revised international standard
series of patch tests" [1]; 34 allergens/test preparations
from three standard series from Europe (EECDRG),
from USA (NACDG), and from Japan (JSDS) were
compared. They were divided in a modified international standard series (20 allergens), and an extended international standard series and additional
useful allergens (8+6, respectively). These 34 aller-
gens/test preparations are reviewed in this booklet.
To aid the reader, we provide an abbreviated exposure sheet which we hope will be of practical value.
The editors welcome comments, additions, correc-
tions, and suggestions for future editions.
We would like to thank all our contributors for their
excellent work.

JAN E. WAHLBERG, PETER ELSNER,
LASSE KANERVA, HOWARD I. MAIBACH,
for the ICDRG

---

[1] Contact Dermatitis (1997) 36: 121–123

Addresses

Editors

WAHLBERG, JAN E.
National Institute for Working Life
113 91 Stockholm
Sweden

ELSNER, PETER
Department of Dermatology
Universitätsklinikum Jena
Erfurter Straße 35
07740 Jena
Germany

KANERVA, LASSE
Institute of Occupational Health
Section of Dermatology
Topeliuksenkatu 41 a
00250 Helsinki
Finland

MAIBACH, HOWARD I.
Department of Dermatology
University of California
San Francisco School of Medicine
San Francisco, CA 94143-0989
USA

Contributors   ALANKO, KRISTIINA
                    Finnish Institute of Occupational Health
                    Topeliuksenkatu 41 aA
                    00250 Helsinki
                    Finland

                    ANDERSEN, KLAUS E.
                    Department of Dermatology
                    Odense University Hospital
                    5000 Odense C
                    Denmark

                    AVNSTORP, CHRISTIAN
                    Klinik for Hudsygdomme
                    Roskildevej 264
                    2610 Rödovre
                    Denmark

                    BRUYNZEEL, DERK P.
                    Department of Dermatology
                    Free University Hospital
                    De Boelelaan 1117
                    1081 HV Amsterdam
                    The Netherlands

                    BRUZE, MAGNUS
                    Department of Occupational
                    and Environmental Dermatology
                    Malmö University Hospital
                    205 02 Malmö
                    Sweden

                    CHOWDHURY, MAHBUB M. U.
                    Department of Dermatology
                    University Hospital of Wales
                    Box 100, Heath Park
                    Cardiff CF14 4XW
                    United Kingdom

FÄRM, GUNILLA
Department of Dermatology
Örebro University Hospital
701 85 Örebro
Sweden

FISCHER, TORKEL
Hensvik 253
760 49 Herräng
Sweden

FLYVHOLM, MARI-ANN
National Institute of Occupational Health
Lersö Parkallé 105
2100 Copenhagen
Denmark

FREEMAN, SUSANNE
Skin and Cancer Foundation
Contact and Occupational Clinic
277 Bourke Street, Darlinghurst
2101 Sydney
Australia

GOH, CHEE LEOK
National Skin Centre (S)
1 Mandalay Road
Singapore 308205
Singapore

GOOSSENS, AN
Department of Dermatology
UZKU Leuven
3000 Leuven
Belgium

GRUVBERGER, BIRGITTA
Department of Occupational
and Environmental Dermatology
Malmö University Hospital
205 02 Malmö
Sweden

GUIN, JERE D.
18 Corporate Hill Drive, Suite 100
Little Rock, AR 72205
USA

HANNUKSELA, MATTI
South Karelia Central Hospital
Laihiankatu 6,
53100 Lappeenranta
Finland

HANSSON, CHRISTER
Department of Dermatology
University Hospital
221 85 Lund
Sweden

HINDSÉN, MONICA
Department of Occupational
and Environmental Dermatology
Malmö University Hospital
205 02 Malmö
Sweden

ISAKSSON, MARLÉNE
Department of Occupational
and Environmental Dermatology
Malmö University Hospital
205 02 Malmö
Sweden

JOLANKI, RIITTA
Finnish Institute of Occupational Health
Topeliuksenkatu 41 aA
00250 Helsinki
Finland

LACHAPELLE, JEAN-MARIE
Department of Dermatology
Louvain University, UCL 3033,
30 Clos Chapelle-aux-Champs
1200 Brussels
Belgium

LIDÉN, CAROLA
Department of Occupational
and Environmental Dermatology
Norrbacka
171 76 Stockholm
Sweden

MAIBACH, HOWARD I.
Department of Dermatology
University of California
San Francisco School of Medicine
San Francisco, CA 94143-0989
USA

MÖLLER, HALVOR
Department of Dermatology
Malmö University Hospital
205 02 Malmö
Sweden

PAULSEN, EVY
Department of Dermatology
Odense University Hospital
5000 Odense C
Denmark

SEIDENARI, STEFANIA
Department of Dermatology
University of Modena
Via del Pozzo 71
41100 Modena
Italy

SHAW, STEPHANIE
Culverton, 110, Wycombe Road
Princes Risborough
Bucks HP27 OEY
United Kingdom

WILKINSON, JOHN
Culverton, 110, Wycombe Road
Princes Risborough
Bucks HP27 OEY
United Kingdom

Contents

Alphabetized Listing of Contents

Recommended Patch-test Concentrations

	Allergen-patch-tape	TRUE test ($\mu g/cm^2$)
Balsam of Peru	25% pet.	800
Benzocaine	5% pet.	
Budesonide	0.01% pet.	2
Cetylstearyl alcohol	20% pet.	
Clioquinol	5% pet.	190 (mix)
Cobalt chloride	1% pet.	20
Colophony	20% pet.	1,200
Diazolidinyl Urea	2% pet.	600
Epoxy resin	1% pet.	50
Ethylenediamine dihydrochloride	1% pet.	50
Formaldehyde	1% aq.	180
Fragrance mix	8% pet.	430
Hydrocortisone-17-butyrate	1% ethanol	25
Imidazolidinyl urea	2% pet.	600
Mercapto mix	1–2% pet.	75
Mercaptobenzothiazole	1–2% pet.	75
Methylchloroisothiazolinone and methylisothiazolinone	0.01–0.02% aq.	4
Methyldibromoglutaronitrile	0.05–0.3% pet.	10
Neomycin sulfate	20% pet.	230

	Allergen-patch tape	TRUE test ($\mu g/cm^2$)
Nickel sulfate	5% pet.	200
Paraben mix	16% pet.	1,000
para-Phenylenediamine free base	1% pet.	90
Potassium dichromate	0.5% pet.	23
Primin	0.01% pet.	
Propylene glycol	5% pet., 20% aq. Not finally stated	
p-Tertiary-butylphenol formaldehyde resin	1% pet.	45
Quaternium 15	1% pet.	100
Sesquiterpene lactone mix	0.1% pet.	
Thimerosal	0.1% pet.	8
Thiuram mix	1% pet.	25
Tixocortol pivalate	0.1% pet.	20
Tosylamide/formaldehyde resin	10% pet.	
Urushiol	0.05–2.5 μg in 5 μl acetone. Open test	
Wool alcohols	30% pet.	1,000

aq. aqueous, *pet.* in petrolatum.

Metals

Cobalt Chloride

TORKEL FISCHER

Designations

INCI Name. Cobalt chloride.
Synonyms. Cobaltous chloride; cobaltous chloride hexahydrate; cobalt dichloride, hexahydrate; cobalt (II) chloride hexahydrate; cobalt blue.
CAS No. 7646-79-9.

Test Preparations

- 1.0% pet. European standard (allergen-patch-tape)
- 0.5% pet. Swedish standard
- 20 μg/cm² (TRUE-test system)

The cobalt chloride patch test is a good indicator of cobalt sensitivity. Cobalt is a strong allergen.

Clinics

Patients allergic to cobalt present clinically with contact dermatitis as a rule, although cases of the following also occur:
- Contact urticaria and systemic urticaria
- Palpebral edema
- Photocontact dermatitis
- Erythema multiforme-like eruptions
- Erosive lichen planus from dental prosthesis
- Ashy dermatosis
- Granulomatous reactions from blue cobaltous aluminate pigment used in tattoos

Occurrence

Cobalt is an essential trace element for humans and part of the vitamin B_{12} complex. It can be detected in minor amounts in soil, water, plants, and animal tissue. Cobalt is found in small quantities in cement (mainly in Europe) and in pottery clay, causing significant sensitization in brick layers and pottery workers. However, exposure to cobalt is often difficult to trace.

Cobalt is a silvery metal with many properties similar to those of iron and nickel. It is a contaminant present in nickel and copper ores and is frequently a minor element in nickel compounds. Cobalt is found in many metal-plated objects, including buckles, buttons, snaps, zippers, and costume jewelry. It is found in plated tool handles, utensils, and keys. Cobalt sulfate, cobalt chloride, and cobalt sulfamate are sometimes used to brighten nickel-plated objects. Present in fertilizers used in agriculture, cobalt sulfate is also used to enrich animal feed. Major industrial use of cobalt is in alloys or as a binder of tungsten and other carbides in the production of hard metal. Cobalt is present together with iron, nickel, chromium, and molybdenum in various magnets and high-temperature, high-strength, surgical implant and dental alloys. Cobalt is present in welding rods and occurs in the smoke from welding stainless steel. Organic cobalt compounds are used in adhesives for bonding the brass-plated steel to rubber in steel-braced radial tires and for hydrotreating and desulfurizing in the oil industry. Cobalt is used as an oxidizing agent in automobile exhaust control.

Oxides of cobalt mixed and calcined with other oxides are used to provide blue-green and yellow colors to ceramics, glass, and paints; these colors are also sometimes used in tattoos. The surface of pottery treated with cobalt dyes releases cobalt. Cobalt salts, especially naphtenate, oleate, and linoleate are used as dryers in oil-based paints, lacquers, varnishes, printing inks, and enamels. These salts are also used as pigments in light-brown hair dyes and makeup. Solid soaps may contain cobalt.

Cobalt is present in lamp filaments and is sometimes present in adhesives and certain brands of electronic recording tapes. Cobalt is used as catalyst for the production of terephthalate plastics or as a catalyst or accelerator of polyester and acrylate resin systems and such plastic material may release cobalt.

Products to Avoid   Avoid the following:
- Metallic cobalt in direct contact with the skin
  Nickel-plated objects such as buckles, buttons, snaps, zippers, and costume jewelry often contain cobalt, as do coins
- Ear-piercing using nickel-plated earrings
- Tattoos with dyes containing cobalt salts
- Cobalt-alloyed partial dentures
  Stomatitis has been reported from dentures alloyed with cobalt

Check the label for cobalt in cosmetics such as antiperspirants, makeup, and brown hair dyes.

Avoid work exposure from:
- Metallic dust and cobalt etching in hard metal manufacturing
- Metal salts of electroplating
- Wet cement and wet alkaline clay containing cobalt
- Paints, lacquers, varnishes, printing inks, and enamels containing cobalt
- Animal feed enriched with cobalt salts

Reactions of delayed tuberculin type from injection of vitamin B_{12} in cobalt-allergic individuals. Reactions from orthopedic implants are rare.
Cobalt from ingested food may cause exacerbation of dermatitis. The removal of cobalt-releasing dental braces and dietary restrictions may help extremely sensitive patients.

Cross-reactivity   Cobalt sensitivity is reported more frequently in
                        nickel-allergic patients, and nickel sensitivity is more
                        common in individuals with cobalt allergy. Cobalt
                        allergy also has an association with chromate. It is
                        not known whether these simultaneous patch test
                        reactions are a manifestation of cross-reactivity or
                        are the result of the simultaneous presence of the
                        metals in alloys.

Alternatives   Persons sensitive to cobalt should use plastic or gold
                        instead of metallic cobalt and nickel objects in direct
                        contact with the skin. Sterling silver and platinum
                        can also be used. Clothing with nonmetallic zippers
                        and fasteners can be worn. Metallic items difficult to
                        avoid such as keys may be coated with several layers
                        of clear nail polish; select scissors and tools with
                        handles of plastic or high-quality stainless steel.
                        Liquid soaps provide an alternative to solid soaps.

References

1. Cronin E (1980) Contact dermatitis. Churchill Livingstone,
    Edinburgh, pp 313–326
2. Rietschel RL, Fowler JF Jr (2001) Fisher's contact dermatitis.
    Lippincott Williams and Wilkins, Philadelphia, pp 626–631

Nickel Sulfate

Carola Lidén

Designations

INCI Name. Nickel sulfate.
Synonym. Single nickel salt.
CAS No. 10101-97-0.

Test Preparations

- 5% pet. European standard (allergen-patch-tape)
- 200 µg/cm² (TRUE-test system)

Occurrence

Nickel is a metal used in many alloys, platings, and chemical compounds. Nickel ions are released from several nickel-containing materials when in contact with the skin, owing to the corrosive effect of sweat. High nickel release is seen from nickel silver (German silver), copper-nickel, nickel-brass, some white gold alloys, and from nickel-plated items. Most stainless steels, e.g., 18/8, contain nickel; however, generally it is not released at skin contact. Nickel occurs naturally in food. Alloys for orthopedic implants and dental braces often contain nickel, but most nickel-sensitive persons do not need to avoid such exposure.

From 2001, the EU Nickel Directive limits nickel in items intended for direct and prolonged contact with the skin such as jewelry, watches, buttons, and spectacle frames. The limit value for nickel release is 0.5 µg/cm² per week. The nickel content in piercing posts has to be below 0.05%. Such products will hopefully, in the future, cause less nickel dermatitis. Nickel is not restricted in other types of items.

Products to Avoid   A wide range of items in personal and occupational
use release nickel ions, which may contribute to der-
matitis. It is, however, often difficult to know what
to avoid contact with and how careful to be. It is not
necessary to avoid contact with all metallic items.
A screening test for nickel release (nickel test,
dimethylglyoxime [DMG] test, Fisher test) is simple
to use. Release of nickel ions is indicated by a red or
pink color (positive DMG test) after rubbing the
surface with a cotton wool-tipped stick soaked with
two drops of DMG and ammonia.
It is wise for everybody to avoid direct and prolonged
contact with personal items such as the following, if
they release nickel: jewelry, buttons, zips, watches,
spectacle frames, buckles, hooks, hair pins. People
with nickel allergy and hand eczema should avoid
prolonged or repeated contact with items such as the
following, if they release nickel: tools, scissors, handles, keys, coins, pens, needles, musical instruments,
surgical instruments, electronic chips, taps, pipes,
and other equipment. It may be of benefit for people
with nickel allergy and persistent dermatitis to avoid
also more transient skin contact with items that release nickel.

Cross-reactivity   Simultaneous patch-test reactivity to cobalt chloride
and/or to potassium dichromate is often recorded in
nickel-sensitive persons, who may need to avoid such
exposure. Patch-test reactivity to palladium chloride
in nickel-sensitive persons is due to cross-reactivity,
while the need to avoid exposure is controversial.

Alternatives   High-quality stainless steels such as 18/8 are generally safe at skin contact. Chromium, iron, copper, silver,
gold, aluminum, brass, titanium, etc are other metals
and alloys which, as such, generally do not contain
or release nickel. However, items are often made of
several materials in combination, some of which may

release nickel. Plastic and wood are other alternatives.

The DMG test is useful for indicating items with low nickel release (no pink color). Limitations of the test are, however, that it sometimes may be falsely negative or difficult to interpret due to discoloration. Protective coatings on the surface may be abraded due to wear.

References

1. Andersen K, White IR, Goossens A (2001) Allergens from the standard series. In: Rycroft RJG, Menné T, Frosch PJ, Lepoittevin J-P (eds) Textbook of contact dermatitis, 3rd edn, chap 31. Springer, Heidelberg, pp 611–615
2. Lidén C, Bruze M, Menné T (2001) Metals. In: Rycroft RJG, Menné T, Frosch PJ, Lepoittevin J-P (eds) Textbook of contact dermatitis, 3rd edn, chap 41. Springer, Heidelberg, pp 938–950
3. Lidén C (2000) Nickel. In: Kanerva L, Elsner P, Wahlberg JE, Maibach HI (eds) Handbook of occupational dermatology, chap 66. Springer, Heidelberg, pp 524–533

Potassium Dichromate

CHRISTIAN AVNSTORP

Designations	**INCI Name.** Potassium dichromate. **Synonyms.** Chromates; chromium compounds; chromium salts. **CAS No.** 7778-50-9.
Test Preparations	• 0.5% pet. European standard (allergen-patch-tape) • 23 µg/cm² (TRUE-test system) The test result may be of an irritant nature. This may be one explanation why it is not always possible to locate exposure.
Occurrence	Professional exposure: • Building industries using cement products • Metal and machine works when cutting and using oils • Chromium plating and galvanizing • Tanning industry • Offset printing and lithography Domestic/consumer exposure: • Leather dressings (shoes especially) • Cleaning products (bleaches/detergents) • Makeup
Products to Avoid	Avoid the following products: • Chromium-tanned leather • Wood preservatives • Textile dyes

Avoid work exposure from:
- Wet cement, mortar, concrete, epoxy fillers (often added to cement)
- Well-used cutting and machine oils
- Laboratory test substances
- Photographic chemicals

Alternatives

Use chromate-reduced cement products for mortar and concrete (ferrous sulfate added during production). Change oil for machines more often. Use vegetable-tanned leather shoes or plastic shoes.

References

1. Lidén C, Bruze M, Menné T (2001) Metals. In: Rycroft RJG, Menné T, Frosch PJ, Lepoittevin JP (eds) Textbook of contact dermatitis, 3rd edn. Springer, Berlin, Heidelberg New York, pp 933–980
2. Avnstorp C (2000) Cement. In: Kanerva L, Elsner P, Wahlberg JE, Maibach HI (eds) Handbook of occupational dermatology. Springer, Berlin, Heidelberg New York, pp 556–561

Rubber Chemicals

Thiuram Mix, Mercapto Mix, and Mercaptobenzothiazole

CHRISTER HANSSON

Designations

Synonyms. Tetramethylthiuram monosulfide (TMTM), thiram; tetramethylthiuram disulfide (TMTD); tetraethylthiuram disulfide (TETD), disulfiram; dipentamethylenethiuram disulfide (PTD); 2-mercaptobenzothiazole (2-MBT); dibenzothiazyl disulfide (MBTS); 2-(4-morfolinyl mercapto) benzothiazole (MOR, MBS, MMBT); N-cyclohexyl-2-benzothiazyl sulfenamide (CBS); (and others).

Test Preparations

Thiuram mix: TMTM, TMTD, TETD, PTD:
- 1% pet. European standard (allergen-patch-tape)
- 25 µg/cm² (TRUE-test system)

Mercapto mix: 2-MBT, MBTS, MOR, CBS:
- 2% pet. European standard (allergen-patch-tape)
- 1% pet. International standard (allergen-patch-tape)
- 75 µg/cm² (TRUE-test system)

2-MBT:
- 2% pet. European standard (allergen-patch-tape)
- 1% pet. International standard (allergen-patch-tape)
- 75 µg/cm² (TRUE-test system)

Occurrence

The components of the thiuram mix and the mercapto mix are all used as accelerators in the vulcanization process during rubber production [1]. The accelerators are added to catalyze the cross-binding between the rubber polymers. Different accelerators are added depending on which type of rubber product is produced. A consequence of this is that thiurams are more related to rubber-glove dermatitis and mercaptobenzothiazoles more to shoe dermatitis. In many rubber processes, however, several different accelerators are used together. For that reason there is justification for testing as many as eight rubber accelerators routinely in the standard test series, and often a special rubber series has to be added.

In more than 50% of patients with sensitivity to rubber chemicals, occupational exposure is the major factor [2]. In this group, sensitization through the use of rubber gloves is the reason in 84%. Other rubber products related to occupational dermatitis are rubber boots, rubber grips of tools, cable material, and tires. Among patients with nonoccupational exposure, mostly clothing such as shoes, boots, socks, stockings, and waistbands are suspected. In health care, many products besides gloves are made of rubber, such as tubes, bandages, catheters, condoms, and so on.

Thiurams are the most important rubber allergens. They can be found in essentially all types of rubber products, and the use of thiurams in the production of rubber gloves is one main reason for sensitization to thiurams. There is a tendency today to replace thiurams with dithiocarbamates in gloves in order to minimize the risk of sensitization [3]. The exclusion of dithiocarbamates from the standard series can be questioned from that point of view and complementary dithiocarbamate tests may be necessary.

Thiurams are also present in numerous rubber products besides gloves, such as seals and tubes. The majority of sensitized patients do not work in the rubber industry but rather in manufacturing industries such as car factories and also in health care.

Thiuram-containing rubber products are ubiquitous, and also in office work, for example, there are products with thiurams such as rubber bands.

TETD is also used as an alcohol deterrent (Antabus) and in an emulsion for the treatment of scabies. Thiurams and also dithiocarbamates have fungicide effects and for that reason they are used in agriculture and also in adhesives, paints, and veterinary medications.

Mercaptobenzothiazoles are common accelerators used in most types of rubber production. Their use in the production of gloves has declined due to the risk of sensitization. However, they are still often used in the production of shoes, and MBT sensitivity is one of the most common reasons for shoe dermatitis. Like thiurams, mercaptobenzothiazoles are also used as fungicides in agriculture and in adhesives and paints. They are also a component of some anti-freeze products, cutting oils, and veterinarian products.

Cross-reactivity

Thiurams. The most important concomitant reactive compounds with thiurams are dithiocarbamates (DTCs). Thiurams and dithiocarbamates form a chemical redox pair, which means that they can be converted into each other by oxidizing and reducing substances which may be present normally in the skin. This phenomenon has been shown by registration of concomitant positive patch test reactions in many patients, although not in all. The nature of the redox equilibrium in the skin is not known, but the presence of iron ions facilitates the oxidation of dithiocarbamates to thiurams [4]. Some fungicides are iron-DTC complexes; these are rapidly converted into the corresponding thiurams under physiological conditions. However, DTCs used as rubber accelerators are usually DTC complexes with zinc or manganese ions. These complexes are much more stable, and it is not known whether they are oxidized by endogenous iron to thiurams. On the other hand, thiurams are rapidly reduced by glutathione into dithiocarbamates. We do not know today which substance is the true hapten that mediates the allergy.

Mercaptobenzothiazoles. In a retrospective study on 2,231 patients, 2.4% showed positive patch test reactions to MBT mix [5]. One-half of these patients reacted to all four components of the MBT mix when these were tested as single substance tests, and as many as 75% reacted to the 2-MBT test. The authors proposed the use of only 2-MBT, omitting MBT mix in the standard series. Their results are in accordance with the chemical investigation of the interconversion of MBT compounds [6]. In this study a redox equilibrium between 2-MBT and MBTS was shown, and in the presence of glutathione all compounds of the MBT mix were rapidly converted into 2-MBT, especially if any 2-MBT was present from the beginning as in the MBT mix. However, we do not know whether specific sensitivities to other substances of the MBT mix exist, nor we do know the details of the redox equilibrium. Until that is known, it may be wise to test the components of the MBT mix as single substance tests if more specific analysis is wanted.

Alternatives

Many rubber products are produced in distant foreign countries, and information about the accelerators used can be impossible to obtain. Nonrubber alternatives are usually recommended, but also in synthetic nonrubber products the same accelerators as in products of natural rubber can be used. In health care and especially with regard to gloves, it is reasonable to demand complete information about the accelerators that have been used. This information is always given by serious suppliers. Some of this information can also be found in the literature, and clinics handling patients with occupational dermatoses should carry this information for the gloves that they commonly use. If a sensitivity is discovered to one accelerator, the patient only has to change to gloves of another brand without this accelerator. In this context, it should be mentioned that the term "hypoallergenic" means different things to different suppliers and should for that reason not be used.

References

1. Belsito DV (2000) Rubber. In: Kanerva L, Elsner P, Wahlberg JE, Maibach HI (eds) Handbook of occupational dermatology, Springer, Berlin Heidelberg New York, pp 701–718
2. Hintzenstern J v, Heese A, Koch HU, Peters K-P, Hornstein OP (1991) Frequency, spectrum and occupational relevance of type IV allergies to rubber chemicals. Contact Dermatitis 24:244–252
3. Knudsen BB, Hametner C, Seycek O, Heese A, Koch H-U, Peters K-P (2000) Allergologically relevant rubber accelerators in single-use medical gloves. Contact Dermatitis 43:9–15
4. Bergendorff O, Hansson C (2002) The spontaneous formation of thiuram disulfides in solutions of iron(III) dithiocarbamates. J Agric Food Chem 50:1092–1096
5. Geier J, Gefeller O (1995) Sensitivity of patch tests with rubber mixes: results of the Information Network of Departments of Dermatology from 1990 to 1993. Am J Contact Dermat 6:143–149
6. Hansson C, Agrup G (1993) Stability of the mercaptobenzothiazole compounds. Contact Dermatitis 28:29–34

Preservatives

Diazolidinyl Urea, Imidazolidinyl Urea, and Quaternium 15

JOHN WILKINSON, STEPHANIE SHAW

Diazolidinyl Urea

Designations

INCI Name. Diazolidinyl urea.
Synonym. Germal 11.
CAS No. 78491-02-8.

Test Preparations

- 2% pet. European standard (allergen-patch-tape)
- 600 µg/cm² (TRUE-test system)

Diazolidinyl urea is used as a bactericide. It is a formaldehyde-releasing agent, though neither its bactericidal action nor its allergenicity depends upon the release of formaldehyde.

Occurrence

The main use of diazolidinyl urea is as a preservative in personal care products, more usually cosmetics, and it will appear as diazolidinyl urea on the list of ingredients.

Products to Avoid

Avoid personal care products that have diazolidinyl urea and imidazolidinyl urea on the ingredient list or any product that is unlabelled. Products that were once tolerated may cause reactions due to change of formulation involving a different preservative, even though they may have the same name and packaging. Therefore each new purchase must be checked.

Cross-reactivity

Patients are often also allergic to imidazolidinyl urea, and it seems that sensitivity to diazolidinyl

urea may be a marker for both chemicals, as patients
may have problems related to use of a product containing imidazolidinyl urea and yet may only have
a positive patch test to diazolidinyl urea. They may
also be allergic to formaldehyde and to other
formaldehyde-releasing biocides. Patients who are
formaldehyde-sensitive may be, or may become,
allergic to other formaldehyde-releasing agents.

Alternatives   Use products that have biocides and preservatives
                   that are not related to formaldehyde-releasers. These
                   include: parabens, phenoxyethanol, methylchloro-
                   isothiazolinone and methylisothiazolinone, methyl-
                   dibromoglutaronitrile, and iodopropylbutylcarba-
                   mate.

Imidazolidinyl urea

Designations   **INCI Name.** Imidazolidinyl urea.
                   Synonym. Germal 115.
                   CAS No. 39236-46-9.

Test Preparations • 2% pet. European standard (allergen-patch-tape)
                   • 600 µg/cm² (TRUE-test system)
                   Imidazolidinyl urea is used as a bactericide. It is a
                   formaldehyde-releasing agent, though neither its
                   bactericidal action nor its allergenicity depends
                   upon the release of formaldehyde.

Occurrence   Its main use is as a preservative in personal care
                   products, more usually cosmetics, and it will appear
                   as imidazolidinyl urea on the list of ingredients.
                   Products that were once tolerated may cause reac-
                   tions due to change of formulation involving a dif-
                   ferent preservative, even though they may have the
                   same name and packaging. Therefore each new
                   purchase must be checked. It is also used as a biocide

and bactericide in aqueous household products such as surface- and window-cleaning products.

Products to Avoid   Avoid personal care products that have imidazolidinyl urea and diazolidinyl urea on the ingredient list or any product that is unlabelled. Products for household use are not yet labelled. Therefore if there is a suspicion that a household product is linked to worsening of dermatitis in a imidazolidinyl urea-allergic patient, then the manufacturer will have to be contacted for specific advise.

Cross-reactivity   Patients allergic to imidazolidinyl urea may also be allergic to diazolidinyl urea, formaldehyde, and to other formaldehyde-releasing biocides. Patients who are formaldehyde-sensitive may be, or may become, allergic to imidazolidinyl urea and other formaldehyde-releasing agents.

Alternatives   Use products that have biocides and preservatives that are not related to formaldehyde-releasers. These include: parabens, phenoxycthanol, methylchloro-isothiazolinone and methylisothiazolinone, methyl dibromoglutaronitrile, iodopropylbutylcarbamate.

Quaternium 15

Designations   INCI Name. Quaternium 15.
Synonyms. Dowicil 200; Dowicil 150; Dowicil 75.
CAS No. 4081-31-3.
The chemical name is *cis*-1-(3 chloroallyl)-3,5,7-triaza-1-azoniaddamantane chloride.

Test Preparations   • 1% pet. (allergen-patch-tape)
• 100 µg/cm^2 (TRUE-test system)

Occurrence

Its main use is as a preservative in personal care products, more usually cosmetics, and it will appear as quaternium 15 on the list of ingredients. It is also used as a biocide in household and industrial products, listed as Dowicil 150 and Dowicil 75. These products are used in adhesives, aqueous preservation, construction, ink solutions, latex emulsions, mineral slurries, oil fields, paint, paper pulp, and textiles.

Products to Avoid

Avoid personal care products that have quaternium 15 on the ingredient list or any product that is un-labelled. Products that were once tolerated may cause reactions due to change of formulation involving a different preservative, even though they may have the same name and packaging. Therefore each new purchase must be checked. Products for household and industrial use are not yet labelled. Therefore if there is a suspicion that a household or industrial product is linked to worsening of dermatitis in a quaternium 15-allergic patient, then the manufacturer will have to be contacted for specific advise.

Cross-reactivity

Patients allergic to quaternium 15 may also be allergic to formaldehyde and to other formaldehyde-releasing biocides. Patients who are formaldehyde-sensitive may be, or may become, allergic to quaternium 15 and other formaldehyde-releasing agents. The formaldehyde release from quaternium 15 is dependent upon pH and temperature.

Alternatives

Use products that have biocides and preservatives that are not related to formaldehyde-releasers. These include: parabens, phenoxyethanol, methylchloro-isothiazolinone and methylisothiazolinone, methyl dibromoglutaronitrile, iodopropylbutylcarbamate.

References

1. Jacobs M-C, White IR, Rycroft RJG, Taub N (1995) Patch testing with preservatives at St John's from 1982–1993. Contact Dermatitis 3:247–254
2. Schnuch A, Geier J, Uter W, Frosch PJ (1998) Patch testing with preservatives, antimicrobials and industrial biocides. Results from a multicenter study. Br J Dermatol 138:467–476
3. Perrenoud D, Bircher A, Hunziker T et al. (1994) Frequency of sensitisation to 13 common preservatives in Switzerland. Contact Dermatitis 30:276–279
4. Wilkinson JD, Shaw S, Andersen KE, et al. (2002) Monitoring preservative sensitivity in Europe: a 10-year multicenter study. Contact Dermatitis 46:207–210

Formaldehyde

MARI-ANN FLYVHOLM

Designations

INCI Name. Formaldehyde.
Synonyms. Formalin; formic aldehyde; formol; methanal; methyl aldehyde; methylene oxide; oxomethane; oxymethylene; paraform; CH_2O; HCHO (and others).
CAS No. 50-00-0.

Test Preparations

- 1% formaldehyde aq. (allergen-patch-tape)
- 180 µg formaldehyde/cm^2 (TRUE-test system)

Occurrence

Formaldehyde is a simple, commonly utilized chemical. It occurs both naturally and "man made" in a variety of manufacturing processes and in finished products. Pure formaldehyde (HCHO) is a gas at room temperature. Formaldehyde is highly soluble in water and is commercially available as a 37–40% aqueous solution (formalin) stabilized with methanol (5–35%) to prevent polymerization.

Formaldehyde can occur in chemical products as a component added in the manufacturing process or as a component added to raw materials. Some components can release formaldehyde as part of their function in the products, i.e., formaldehyde-releasing preservatives. Besides these intentional occurrences of formaldehyde, it can occur as residues from synthesis of other components and from formation during storage and handling of raw materials or end products. Contamination from packages coated with formaldehyde resins has also been reported.

Formaldehyde and formaldehyde releasers are used as preservatives in a wide range of products. For industrial purposes it is mainly used in organic synthesis, in the manufacture of plastic products and in the manufacture of resins used in the production of, e.g., particle board, plywood, and foam insulation. Formaldehyde is also used as a disinfectant in the medical field.

According to the European Union (EU) rules for cosmetics, concentrations below 0.2% free formaldehyde are permitted in cosmetic products (0.1% in products for oral hygiene), and the limit for labeling with the warning "contains formaldehyde" is 0.05%. According to new EU rules for chemical products, formaldehyde content above 0.2% requires labeling with risk-phrase R43: "May cause sensitization by skin contact".

Products to Avoid   Studies on exposure to formaldehyde in patients with contact dermatitis and sensitivity to formaldehyde have shown that products containing formaldehyde-releasing preservatives are frequent sources of formaldehyde exposure.

The release of formaldehyde in products that contain formaldehyde-releasing preservatives cannot be predicted from the formulation. Thus, for treatment purposes it is most convenient to regard all products containing formaldehyde or formaldehyde releasers as sources of formaldehyde exposure and advise patients to use alternative products if possible.

Formaldehyde and/or formaldehyde-releasing preservatives may occur in a wide range of products for personal, household, or occupational use. A list of products containing formaldehyde or formaldehyde-releasing preservatives cannot be expected to be exhaustive and will be outdated quickly. More important than listing products or product types is the point that patients and clinicians should examine a current and updated product declaration when deciding whether or not a product is safe to use.

Formaldehyde has been reported in a wide range of products such as:
- Adhesives/glues
- Cleaning agents
- Building materials
- Corrosion inhibitors
- Filling agents
- Flooring agents
- Hardeners
- Impregnating agents,
- Paints/lacquers
- Metalworking and cutting fluids
- Printing inks
- Polishes

and in raw materials such as:
- Binding agents
- Coloring agents
- Surface active agents

Formaldehyde-releasing preservatives are frequently used in cosmetics, skin care products such as creams, and personal care products such as shampoos, soaps, and skin cleansers. Among household and occupationally used products, formaldehyde-releasing preservatives may occur in, for example, adhesives/glues, cleaning agents, dishwashing liquids, impregnating agents, metalworking and cutting fluids, paints/lacquers, and polishes.

Uses of formaldehyde resins, relevant for skin exposure, are used as textile finishing for permanent-press and waterproof fabrics. In some countries regulations set limitations for formaldehyde in textiles and clothes. Formaldehyde resins may also occur in high-quality paper.

Alternatives

Products which do not contain formaldehyde or formaldehyde-releasing preservatives will normally be safe to use. For cosmetics, personal care products, household products, and occupational products, it is advisable to use products with full product declaration or to contact the supplier or manufacturer and make sure that the product does not contain formaldehyde or formaldehyde releasers. Before purchasing or using a product, the list of ingredients should be checked against a list of formaldehyde-releasing preservatives (see Table 1).

An alternative method for surveying formaldehyde exposure is to use the relatively simple tests methods available for clinical assessment of formaldehyde, i.e., the chromotropic acid test and the acetylacetone test.

References

1. Flyvholm M-A (1997) Formaldehyde exposure at the workplace and in the environment. Allergologie 5:225–231
2. Flyvholm M-A, Andersen P (1993) Identification of formaldehyde releasers and occurrence of formaldehyde and formaldehyde releasers in registered chemical products. Am J Ind Med 24:533–552
3. Flyvholm M-A, Tiedeman E, Menné T (1996) Comparison of 2 tests used for clinical assessment of formaldehyde exposure. Contact Dermatitis 34:35–38

Table 1. Formaldehyde-releasing preservatives, which may cause reactions in patients with contact allergy to formaldehyde. (Adapted from Flyvholm and Andersen 1993 Am J Ind Med 24:533–552)

CAS no.	INCI name	Systematic chemical names	Synonyms
14548-60-8	Benzylhemiformal	(Phenylmethoxy)methanol	Benzylhemiformal Benzyloxymethanol Phenylmethoxymethanol
7747-35-5	7-Ethylbicyclo-oxazolidine	7a-Ethyldihydro-1H,3H, 5H-oxazolo[3,4-c]oxazole	Ethyldihydrooxazolo[3,4-c]oxazole 5-Ethyl-1-aza-3,7-dioxabicyclo[3.3.0]octane
30007-47-7	5-Bromo-5-nitro-1,3-dioxane	5-Bromo-5-nitro-1,3-dioxane	Bromonitrodioxane Bronidox
52-51-7	2-Bromo-2-nitro-propane-1,3-diol	2-Bromo-2-nitro-1,3-propanediol	Bromonitropropanediol Bronopol
4080-31-3 (51229-78-8)	Quaternium-15	N-(3-Chloroallyl)hexamethylene-tetraminiumchloride (the *cis* isomer of this substance)	Chloroallylhexaminium chloride 3-Chloroallyl hexaminium chloride Methenamine 3-chloroallylochloride Dowicil 75 Dowicil 200
78491-02-8	Diazolidinyl urea	N-(1,3-Bis(hydroxymethyl)-2,5-dioxo-4-imidazolidinyl)-N,N'-bis(hydroxymethyl)urea	Tetramethylolhydantoin urea Germall II
109-87-5	Methylal	Dimethoxymethane	Formal Methylal

Table 1 (continued)

CAS no.	INCI name	Systematic chemical names	Synonyms
9065-13-8	DMHF	Formaldehyde, polymer with dimethyl-2,4-imidazolidinedione	Dimethylhydantoin formaldehyde resin
140-95-4	Not available	N,N'-Bis(hydroxymethyl)urea	Dimethylol urea Dihydroxymethylurea
6440-58-0	DMDM hydantoin	1,3-Bis(hydroxymethyl)-5,5-dimethyl-2,4-imidazolidinedione	Dimethyloldimethylhydantoin 1,3-Dimethylol-5,5-dimethylhydantoin DMDMH Glydant
100-97-0	Methenamine	1,3,5,7-Tetraazatricyclo (3.3.1.1^{3,7})decane	Hexamethylenetetramine Hexamine Urotropine
461-72-3	Not available	2,4-Imidazolidinedione	Hydantoin Glycolylurea
39236-46-9	Imidazolidinyl urea	N,N''-Methylenebis(N'-(3-(hydroxymethyl)-2,5-dioxo-4-imidazolidinyl)urea)	Bis(methylolhydantoin urea) methane Germall 115
116-25-6	MDM hydantoin	1-Hydroxymethyl-5,5-dimethyl-2,4-imidazolidinedione	MDM hydantoin Monomethyloldimethylhydantoin MDMH
66204-44-2	Not available	3,3'-Methylenebis(5-methyloxazolidine)	N,N'-Methylenebis(5-methyloxazolidine) Grotan OX

Table 1 (continued)

CAS no.	INCI name	Systematic chemical names	Synonyms
2832-19-1	Not available	2-Chloro-N-(hydroxymethyl)-acetamide	N-Methylolchloracetamide Parmetol K50 Preventol D3 Preventol D5
34375-28-5	Not available	2-(Hydroxymethylamino)ethanol	N-Methylolethanolamine
30525-89-4	Not available	Paraformaldehyde	Polyoxymethylene
4719-04-4	Not available	1,3,5-Triazine-1,3,5(2H,4H,6H)-triethanol	Trihydroxyethylhexahydro-s-triazine Grotan BK KM 200
126-11-4	Tris(hydroxymethyl)nitromethane	2-(Hydroxymethyl)-2-nitro-1,3-propanediol	Trimethylolnitromethane Nitromethylidynetrimethanol

CAS No. Chemical Abstracts Service registry number, *INCI* International Nomenclature of Cosmetic Ingredients.

Methylchloroisothiazolinone and Methylisothiazolinone

BIRGITTA GRUVBERGER

Methylchloroisothiazolinone

Designations   INCI Name. Methylchloroisothiazolinone.
Synonym. 5-Chloro-2-methyl-4-isothiazolin-3-one.
CAS No. 26172-55-4.

Methylisothiazolinone

Designations   INCI Name. Methylisothiazolinone.
Synonym. 2-Methyl-4-isothiazolin-3-one.
CAS No. 2682-20-4.

Methylchloroisothiazolinone and Methylisothiazolinone (3:1) Mixture

Designations   INCI Name. Methylchloroisothiazolinone/
methylisothiazolinone.
Synonyms. Kathon CG; Cl+Me-isothiazolinone;
MCI/MI.
CAS No. 55965-84-9.

Test Preparations   **Allergen-patch-tape.** Two standards are used:
- Mixture in the ratio 3:1 of methylchloroisothiazoli-
  none and methylisothiazolinone 0.01% water w/v
  (Kathon CG)
- Mixture in the ratio 3:1 of methylchloroisothiazolinone and methylisothiazolinone 0.02% water w/v
  (Kathon CG; Swedish standard series)
  The Swedish Contact Dermatitis Group has recommended 0.02%, because dose-response studies
  have indicated that up to 50% of the cases might
  have been missed when tested with 0.01%

TRUE-test System. A mixture in the ratio 3:1 of
methylchloroisothiazolinone and methylisothiazolinone 4 μg/cm^2 (Kathon CG).

Occurrence   Methylchloroisothiazolinone and methylisothiazolinone are active ingredients in many preservatives
marketed under various brand names. Since pure
methylchloroisothiazolinone and methylisothiazolinone are not commercially available, patch testing is
performed with the preservative Kathon CG, containing a mixture in the ratio 3:1 of
methylchloroisothiazolinone and methylisothiazolinone.
Kathon CG became widely used in cosmetic products and toiletries during the 1980s and many reports on contact allergy were published. The mixture
of methylchloroisothiazolinone and methylisothiazolinone has a strong sensitizing potential, and animal studies have demonstrated methylchloroisothiazolinone is a potent sensitizer and methylisothiazolinone a weak sensitizer.
Methylchloroisothiazolinone and methylisothiazolinone can occur in lotions, creams, moisturizers, and
emollients (leave-on products), and shampoos, hair
conditioners, and liquid soaps, etc. (rinse-off products). To prevent sensitization to methylchloroiso-

thiazolinone and methylisothiazolinone, it has been recommended not to use methylchloroisothiazolinone and methylisothiazolinone in leave-on products. Thus, today methylchloroisothiazolinone and methylisothiazolinone are mainly used in rinse-off products.

According to the European legislation, all cosmetic products and toiletries should be supplied with a list of their ingredients using the International Nomenclature of Cosmetic Ingredients (INCI). Thus, if methylchloroisothiazolinone and methylisothiazolinone are ingredients in cosmetic products and toiletries you will find methylchloroisothiazolinone and methylisothiazolinone on the lists.

Preservatives containing methylchloroisothiazolinone and methylisothiazolinone have a broad spectrum of applications among industrial products, since they are effective against bacteria, fungi, yeast, and algae at low concentrations. Some preservatives contain high concentrations of methylchloroisothiazolinone and methylisothiazolinone. They are corrosive and skin exposure can cause chemical burns and induce sensitization. Therefore, patch-testing with Kathon CG is recommended in all individuals with chemical burns caused by preservatives containing methylchloroisothiazolinone and methylisothiazolinone.

Methylchloroisothiazolinone and methylisothiazolinone can be found in paints/lacquers, cleaning agents, printing inks, coloring agents, polish, binding agents, adhesives/glues, filling agents, impregnating agents, metalworking and cutting fluids, fountain water, cooling-tower water, etc.

Previously all preservatives containing methylchloroisothiazolinone also contained methylisothiazolinone, since both were formed during the synthesis. Recently preservatives containing only methylisothiazolinone were introduced on the market. Minimal experience as to its sensitization potential exists.

Products to Avoid   Individuals sensitized to methylchloroisothiazoli-
none/methylisothiazolinone should avoid leave-on
products containing methylchloroisothiazolinone
and methylisothiazolinone. Prolonged skin exposure
to industrial products containing methylchloroisothiazolinone and methylisothiazolinone should be
avoided. Rinse-off products containing methylchloroisothiazolinone and methylisothiazolinone
pose a low risk of skin problems when they are used
on normal skin. However, although no studies have
been performed on the significance of exposure to
methylchloroisothiazolinone and methylisothiazoli-
none-containing rinse-off products on damaged
skin, our patients are advised not to choose these
rinse-off products.

Cross-reactivity   Cross-reactivity between methylchloroisothiazolinone and methylisothiazolinone and the two isothia-
zolinones 1,2-benzisothiazolin-3-one and 2-n-octyl-
4-isothiazolin-3-one have been investigated but no
cross-reactions were shown. 1,2-Benzisothiazolin-3-
one and 2-n-octyl-4-isothiazolin-3-one are biocidal
chemicals intended for industrial products.

Alternatives   Several preservatives are available on the market.
Thus, it should be possible to choose products
containing preservatives other than methylchloroisothiazolinone and methylisothiazolinone.

References   1. Gruvberger B (1998) Methylisothiazolinones. Diagnosis
and prevention of allergic contact dermatitis. Acta Derm
Venereol Suppl (Stockh) 200:1–42
2. Fewings J, Menné T (1999) An update of the risk assessment
for methylchloroisothiazolinone/methylisothiazolinone
(MCI/MI) with focus on rinse-off products. Contact
Dermatitis 41:1–13
3. Reinhard E, Waeber R, Niederer M, Maurer T, Maly P,
Scherer S (2001) Preservation of products with MCI/MI in
Switzerland. Contact Dermatitis 45:257–264

Methyldibromoglutaronitrile

BIRGITTA GRUVBERGER, MAGNUS BRUZE

Designations

INCI Name. Methyldibromoglutaronitrile.
Synonym. 1,2-Dibromo-2,4-dicyanobutane.
CAS No. 35691-65-7.

Test Preparation

Currently, there is no agreement on the optimal test preparation using allergen-patch tape. The following is proposed for a modified international standard series: methyldibromoglutaronitrile 0.1% pet. w/w.

Other available test preparations are:
- Methyldibromoglutaronitrile 0.3% pet. w/w
- Methyldibromoglutaronitrile 0.05% pet. w/w
- Euxyl K400 1.5% pet. w/w
- 10 μg/cm^2 (TRUE-test system)

Occurrence

Euxyl K 400 is a preservative for cosmetic products and toiletries consisting of methyldibromoglutaronitrile and 2-phenoxyethanol in a 1:4 ratio. Euxyl K 400 was introduced on the market as an alternative to the sensitizing methylchloroisothiazolinone/methylisothiazolinone (Kathon CG) partly because of no demonstrable sensitizing capacity in the guinea pig. Euxyl K 400 was demonstrated as a new sensitizer in cosmetics in the early 1990s and was soon proved to be a frequent cause of allergic contact dermatitis from cosmetics. Eventually, animal studies demonstrated methyldibromoglutaronitrile to be a sensitizer. To detect the allergenic property, a predictive test method with multiple topical applications had to be used.

Methyldibromoglutaronitrile can be found in cosmetics, ultrasonic gels, toiletries, moistened toilet tissues, hygienic products, glues, joint fillings, and cleaning agents.

Products to Avoid   Many reports on contact allergy to methyldibromoglutaronitrile have been published. Leave-on products and moistened toilet tissues seem to be the most common sources of sensitization to methyldibromoglutaronitrile. The risks of sensitization and/or elicitation of allergic contact dermatitis from rinse-off products are lower. Consequently, individuals sensitized to methyldibromoglutaronitrile are recommended to avoid leave-on products containing methyldibromoglutaronitrile as well as prolonged skin exposure to industrial products containing methyldibromoglutaronitrile. Concerning rinse-off products containing methyldibromoglutaronitrile, there seems to be a negligible risk of skin problems when they are used on normal skin. However, although no studies have been performed on the significance of exposure to rinse-off products containing methyldibromoglutaronitrile on damaged skin, our patients are advised not to choose rinse-off products containing methyldibromoglutaronitrile.

Cross-reactivity   No cross-reacting substances are known.

Alternatives   Several preservatives are available. Thus, it should be possible to choose products without methyldibromoglutaronitrile.

References

1. Gruvberger B, Bruze M (1997) Preservatives. Clinics in Dermatology. Contact Dermatitis 15:493–497
2. Wahlkvist H, Boman A, Montelius J, Wahlberg JE (1999) Sensitizing potential in mice, guinea pig and man of the preservative Euxyl K 400 and its ingredient methyldibromoglutaronitrile. Contact Dermatitis 41:330–338
3. Tosti A, Vincenzi C, Smith KA (2000) Provocative use testing of methyldibromoglutaronitrile in a cosmetic shampoo. Contact Dermatitis 42:64–67

Parabens

Susanne Freeman

Methylparaben

Designations

INCI Name. Methylparaben.
Synonyms. Methyl 4-hydroxybenzoate; Nipagin M.
CAS No. 99-76-3.

Ethylparaben

Designations

INCI Name. Ethylparaben.
Synonym. Ethyl 4-hydroxybenzoate.

Propylparaben

Designations

INCI Name. Propylparaben.
Synonym. Propyl 4-hydroxybenzoate.
CAS No. 94-13-3.

Butylparaben

Designations

INCI Name. Butylparaben.
Synonym. Butyl 4-hydroxybenzoate.

Test Preparation

- Paraben mix consists of 4% methyl-*p*-hydroxy-benzoate, ethyl-*p*-hydroxy-benzoate, propyl-*p*-hydroxy-benzoate and butyl-*p*-hydroxy-benzoate (total of 16% in pet.)

- 1,000 µg/cm² (TRUE-test system)

The paraben-mixture responses are frequently irritant; positives should be tested to the individual paraben for confirmation.

Occurrence   Parabens are preservatives in cosmetics and medicaments.

Products to Avoid Products containing parabens rarely sensitize, except in patients with stasis dermatitis and leg ulcers. But leg ulcer patients can often use parabens-preserved cosmetics on normal skin without trouble.

Cross-reactivity   Other *para* compounds, e.g., benzocaine, *para*-phenylenediamine, and sulfonamides.

Alternatives   If true allergy to parabens in cosmetics or medicaments is diagnosed, patients must use products containing an alternative preservative.

References
1. Andersen KE, White IR, Goossens A (2001) Allergens from the standard series. In: Rycroft RJG, Menne T, Frosch PJ, Lepoittevin J-P (eds) Textbook of contact dermatitis. Springer, Berlin Heidelberg New York, pp 631–632
2. Uter W, Schnuch A, Geier J, Agathos M (2002) Epikutantest – Reaktionen auf Paraben-Mixe und ihre Aufschlüsselungen. Allergologie 25:194–202

Thimerosal

Halvor Möller

INCI Name. Thimerosal.
Synonyms. Thiomersal; merthiolate; sodium ethyl-mercuric thiosalicylate.
CAS No. 54-64-8.

Test Preparations
- 0.1% pet. (allergen-patch-tape)
- 8 µg/cm² (TRUE-test system)

Occurrence
A preservative formerly incorporated in many creams and solutions for skin care, in eye and ear drops, in cleansing solutions for contact lenses, in disinfectant solutions, in solvents for intra-dermal testing (tuberculin, as well as hay fever and asthma allergens), and in several vaccines. From most of these sources, thimerosal has been removed.
To-day, thimerosal can be found world-wide in vaccines against, e.g., influenza, hepatitis, and tick-borne encephalitis. In some countries, thimerosal solutions are sold over the counter (OTC) for skin disinfection.

Cross-reactivity
Thimerosal is an organic mercury salt but not a marker for contact allergy to mercury. Most studies deny cross-reactivity to metallic and inorganic mercury. The allergenic determinant is the ethylmercury moiety in most cases, the thiosalicylate part in some. In the latter case, there is a concomitant photoallergy

to piroxicam, a nonsteroidal anti-inflammatory drug (NSAID).

Primary Prophylaxis. There is world-wide a paradoxically high frequency of contact allergy to thimerosal in patients with eczematous disease, as well as in healthy populations, but with a very low clinical relevance. A correspondingly high, epicutaneous exposure is not known except in countries where thimerosal-containing disinfectants are sold OTC. Therefore, the source and route of sensitization is not fully understood.

Vaccines are given intramuscularly or subcutaneously, routes that are notoriously poor for inducing contact allergy. Still, some epidemiological data point toward a positive correlation between exposure to thimerosal-containing vaccines and the development of contact allergy to the preservative. However, a prerequisite for sensitization seems to be a leakage of the allergen into the injection canal and deposition close to immunocompetent cells in epidermis and/or dermis. Thus, care should be taken to avoid such contamination during vaccination.

Secondary Prophylaxis. Obviously, allergic subjects should stay away from skin disinfectants containing thimerosal. On the other hand, vaccinations seem to be without risk of eliciting a clinical allergic reaction in subjects already sensitized to thimerosal. The concentration of the preservative in vaccines is very low. Furthermore, experimental as well as clinical studies have shown that parenteral injections of thimerosal-containing vaccines do not lead to rashes or eczematous reactions in the skin, nor to any adverse reactions in other organs. In a few patients, a limited local reaction at the injection site has been registered. Thus, patients with a contact allergy to thimerosal do not need to abstain from vaccinations even if thimerosal is incorporated in the vaccine.

References

1. Möller H (1994) All these positive tests to thimerosal. Contact Dermatitis 31:209–213
2. Suneja T, Belsito DV (2001) Thimerosal in the detection of clinically relevant allergic contact reactions. J Am Acad Dermatol 45:23–27
3. Audicana MT, Munoz D, Pozo MD del, Fernández E, Gastaminza G, Corres LF de (2002) Allergic contact dermatitis from mercury antiseptics and derivatives: study protocol of tolerance to intramuscular injections of thimerosal. Am J Contact Dermatitis 13:3–9

Perfumes and Fragrances

Balsam of Peru (Myroxylon pereirae)

Derk P. Bruynzeel

INCI Name. Myroxylon pereirae.
Synonyms. Balsam of Tolu; Peru balsam; balsam Peru.
CAS No. 8007-00-9.

Test Preparations
- 25.0% pet. (allergen-patch-tape)
- 800 µg/cm² (TRUE-test system)

Occurrence

Balsam of Peru (myroxylon pereirae) is an aromatic resin obtained from the tree *Myroxylon balsamum* (L) *var. pereirae* (Leguminosae) by damaging the tree bark. The tree is a native to Central America and the balsam is currently produced by El Salvador. The balsam has been used as a bactericide in topical medical preparations. It contains many unknown constituents. Important components are: benzoic acid, benzyl benzoate, benzyl cinnamate, cinnamic acid, cinnamyl cinnamate, nerolidol, farnesol, and eugenol. These or closely related chemicals are also found in other balms (balsam of Tolu, styrax, tea-tree oil) and spices such as cinnamon, clove, and nutmeg, and they are used in perfumes. Myroxylon pereirae can be used as a fragrance, although it is not recommended. Balsam of Peru or its constituents may be used in the food industry (e.g., in sweets, chocolate, drinks, liqueurs), the tobacco industry (flavoring of tobacco), and even in some pharmaceutical products (e.g., cough mixtures, suppositories, dental preparations).

Balsam of Peru is used in the contact allergy investigations as a fragrance allergy marker.

Cross-reactivity   Cross-reactivity to a number of chemicals and plant extracts is known to occur:

- Balsam of Tolu
- Styrax
- Tiger balm
- Propolis
- Tea-tree oil
- Colophony
- Wood tars
- Turpentine
- Benzoin
- Benzoic acid
- Benzyl benzoate
- Benzaldehyde
- Benzylsalicylate
- Coniferyl alcohol
- Coumarin
- Eugenol
- Isoeugenol
- Diethylstilbestrol
- Farnesol
- Citrus peel
- Clove
- Nutmeg
- Cinnamon
- Various perfumes

This could be because of close relationship or because the same chemical is also present in the balm.

Products to Avoid   As there is a close relation to fragrance allergy, it is advisable to avoid perfumed products (cosmetics, toiletries) and balms (listed above). It is also an indicator for spices and flavors: skin contact may cause allergic contact dermatitis in those preparing food. Eating may cause a sore mouth, cheilitis, or some-

times a flare-up of the dermatitis elsewhere, for
example on the hands (vesicular dermatitis). The
peel of citrus fruits can be a "hidden" source of
contact.
Sometimes, eating food containing related chemicals
may cause also a flare-up. This does not happen in
many patients, but it is important to remember that
this may be a contact source. Products to be aware of
are: citrus peel (marmalade, juice), bakery products,
candy, chewing gum, tobacco, cough mixtures, cola
and cola-like soft drinks, spices and spicy food,
liqueurs, etc.

Alternatives

Fragrance-free cosmetics and toiletries; see from the
ingredients label of those products whether they
contain fragrance (perfume) or myroxylon pereirae.
Try to avoid mixed spices, unless the ingredients are
specified; be careful with spicy food.
If you want to use a perfumed product try it first in
a repeated open application test (ROAT). Apply the
product twice daily to the antecubital space for
14 days. If no reaction occurs – itching, redness, dermatitis – the product may probably be used without
adverse effects.

References

1. Rietschel RL, Fowler JF (2001) Fisher's contact dermatitis,
   5th edn. Lippincott, Williams and Wilkins, Philadelphia,
   pp 137–140, 363–364
2. Rycroft RJG, Menné T, Frosch PJ, Lepoittevin JP (2001)
   Textbook of contact dermatitis, 3rd edn. Springer, Berlin
   Heidelberg New York, pp 623–625
3. Hjorth N (1961) Eczematous allergy to balsams. Munks-
   gaard, Copenhagen
4. Niinimäki A (1995) Double-blind placebo-controlled peroral
   challenges in patients with delayed-type allergy to balsam
   of Peru. Contact Dermatitis 33:78–83

Fragrance Mix

DERK P. BRUYNZEEL

Designations

INCI Names, Synonyms, and CAS Nos. Oak moss; isoeugenol (97-54-1); eugenol (97-53-0); cinnamal (cinnamic aldehyde; 104-55-2); geraniol (106-24-1); hydroxycitronellal (laurine; 107-75-5); cynamyl alcohol (cinnamic alcohol; 104-54-1); cinnamic aldehyde (alpha-amyl cinnamic aldehyde; 122-40-7).

Test Preparations

- 1% pet. for each fragrance allergen
  The mix may contain sorbitan sesquioleate (concentration 5%), an emulsifier which enhances the diagnostic value of the mix (original patch-test system)
- 430 µg/cm^2 (350 µg/patch), equal amounts (weight) for each allergen (TRUE-test system)

The fragrance mix consists of eight common fragrances. A positive patch test reaction to the fragrance mix indicates a perfume allergy, or at least a contact sensitization to one or more of the fragrance allergens in the mix. The ingredients of the mix represent the most commonly involved fragrance allergens. Fragrance allergy is common; reported prevalence rates vary between 5 and 12%. Testing with mixes has some problems; there is a chance that false positive reactions will be induced. This also occurs to some degree with the fragrance mix. On the other hand, false negatives occur as well. If doubt arises about the test results, it is important

to repeat the test procedure for each of the individual ingredients of the mix. The ingredients can
be tested separately at a higher concentration, usually 2%.

Occurrence   A perfume is a complex product usually containing
                    many, sometimes more than 100, ingredients. Not all
                    ingredients are known sensitizers. The ingredients of
                    the fragrance mix are, however, essential for most
                    perfumes. Some are synthetic chemicals, others are
                    obtained from plant extracts, including lavender,
                    jasmine, rose, sandalwood, ylang-ylang, and balsam
                    of Peru.
                    Fragrances are found in perfumes, toilet water, and
                    colognes; but cosmetics and toiletries usually also
                    contain perfume: creams, milks, lotions, lipsticks,
                    eye-cosmetics, powders, soaps, shampoos, and
                    shower and bath products. The content of the ingre-
                    dients of cosmetics is written on the package or the
                    container. Fragrances or perfumes are mentioned as
                    such and not (yet) the individual components, so it
                    is possible to identify the products that contain per-
                    fume. Some cosmetics are not scented and often
                    these products are labeled "fragrance free". However,
                    one should be careful, as nonperfumed products may
                    contain a low concentration of a masking fragrance
                    to cover an unpleasant smell of some of the other
                    chemicals in the product. Another problem may be
                    the incorporation of an essential oil, for example
                    rose oil, or just a single fragrance chemical. These
                    may not be recognized on the ingredient list as a
                    fragrance by the patient.
                    Many household products for cleaning and washing
                    contain perfumes. Sometimes perfumes are added to
                    the air in ventilation systems in buildings and air-
                    planes. In the same category fall the use (burning) of
                    fragranced wax candles and incense. Aromatherapy
                    is another source which might be overlooked.

Unexpected sources of perfumed products may range from sanitary towels, tissues, toilet paper, and industrial products such as metal-working fluids. Sometimes even topical medical preparations contain a fragrance.

Another source of fragrances can be found in spices and seasonings. Spices such as cinnamon contain essential oils which are also used in perfumes. Skin contact with such spices and seasonings can thus cause contact allergic reactions. Consuming spices usually does not cause problems.

Products to Avoid

The advice "avoid perfumed products" is simple but in practice difficult, as so many products contain a perfume while only a few groups of products are labeled as such. Cosmetics used by a partner may be an overlooked source. Cosmetics and toiletries do have ingredient labeling but may contain fragrance allergens which might be overlooked as they are not recognized as fragrance.

Wash-off cosmetics such as shampoo and soap do not always cause allergic reactions in sensitized persons because of the short contact and the low perfume concentrations. Stay-on products are more likely to cause trouble.

Balms such as balsam of Peru, tiger balsam, propolis, tea-tree oil and colophony should be avoided.

Those who have a fragrance allergy and do have skin contact (preparing food) with spices and seasonings should avoid skin contact, as the essential oils of these materials are related to many fragrances. Eating of these materials will sometimes cause a flare-up of the eczema; however, this is not common.

Cross-reactivity

Fragrance chemicals can be closely related and thus cross-react. More of a problem is that many "natural" and "herbal" products used for personal care are promoted as healthy products that are not harmful.

Yet they contain oils and ingredients that are related to the well-known fragrance allergens. Balms such as balsam of Peru, tiger balsam, propolis, and tea-tree oil often fall into this category. Colophony, for example in cosmetics (pressed powders), may cross-react.

Alternatives

Alternatives are nonscented products. Cosmetics and toiletries labeled "fragrance free" are usually reliable. Sometimes wash-off products such as soap are tolerated if the skin is well rinsed after use. Perfume applied to a piece of material and pinned under the sleeve of a blouse may be a help for those who want to use a perfume.

Repeated Open Application Test. A ROAT is advised for those who still want to try a scented product. Apply the product that you want to use twice daily up to 14 days to the antecubital space. A lack of reaction, itch, redness, or dermatitis, suggests that the product can be used without adverse effects.

References

1. De Groot A, Frosch P (1997) Adverse reactions to fragrances. Contact Dermatitis 36:57–86
2. Rietschel RL, Fowler JF (2001) Fisher's contact dermatitis. Lippincott, Williams and Wilkins, Philadelphia, pp 343–350
3. Rycroft RJG, Menné T, Frosch PJ, Lepoittevin JP (2001) Textbook of contact dermatitis, 3rd edn. Springer, Berlin Heidelberg New York, pp 619–623

Corticosteroids

Budesonide, Tixocortol Pivalate, and Hydrocortisone-17-Butyrate

Marléne Isaksson

Corticosteroids can be classified into four groups according to their allergenicity: groups A, B, C, and D1/D2 [1, 2]. Members of a group have the potential to cross-react with each other, whereas cross-reactions between groups are not typically seen. One exceptions is budesonide, which cross-reacts not only with corticosteroids of the acetonide group (group B), to which it belongs, but also with members of group D2 due to its S-isomer. Similarly hydrocortisone-17-butyrate from group D2 may cross-react with budesonide through its S-isomer.

The metabolization of corticosteroids in the skin can also lead to cross-reactions between some classes, if the molecules behave as haptens before and after biometabolization. One example is hydrocortisone-17-butyrate (group D2), which is converted to hydrocortisone-21-butyrate and then further enzymatically converted to hydrocortisone (group A). Other examples are methylprednisolone aceponate (group D2) which is converted via several steps to methylprednisolone (group A), and prednicarbate (group D2) to prednisolone (group A). This means, that corticosteroids from group A may cross-react with corticosteroids from group D2, and corticosteroids from group D2 may cross-react with corticosteroids from group A.

Markers for group A and B corticosteroids should be present in any standard series to detect cortico-

steroid allergy [3]. The patch-test readings should be
performed on day 3 or 4 and on day 7, because corticosteroid allergy may be missed if late readings are
not done [4]. A dermatitis patient should be patch-
tested not only with the group A and B markers of
corticosteroid allergy, but also with the different corticosteroids used by the patient (the pure corticosteroid in an appropriate vehicle and concentration).
In the UK, betamethasone valerate and clobetasol
propionate are widely used and patients sensitized to
them are not identified with the markers for groups
A and B [5]. This kind of testing also pertains to
patients with corticosteroid-treated asthma/rhinitis
and to patients having taken systemic corticosteroids, in case a corticosteroid allergy type IV is
suspected [6, 7]. If a corticosteroid allergy is found,
an extended corticosteroid series should be tested
not to miss other contact allergies and to detect
cross-reactions, so that further treatment and appropriate information regarding local as well as systemic therapy may be given.

Budesonide

Designations	**INCI Name.** Budesonide.
	CAS No. 51333-22-3.
Test Preparation	• 0.01% pet. (allergen-patch-tape)
Occurrence	Budesonide is a screening agent for corticosteroid sensitivity and a marker for group B corticosteroids. It is a potent corticosteroid still present in some topical pharmaceuticals intended for the treatment of corticosteroid-responsive diseases, above all skin diseases. Budesonide is also used in various nasal and pulmonary medicaments to treat rhinitis, asthma, and chronic lung diseases. It may also be

present in tablets to make a rectal suspension for the treatment of various kinds of colitis and proctitis and as capsules to be taken orally in the treatment of Crohn's disease.

Products to Avoid Topical, nasal, pulmonary, rectal, and oral pharmaceuticals containing budesonide. Also, medicaments containing potentially cross-reacting corticosteroids should be avoided. These may be used in topical as well as systemic treatments.

Cross-reactivity Corticosteroids belonging to group B corticosteroids should be avoided:
- Amcinonide
- Desonide
- Flucloronide
- Flunisolide
- Fluocinolone acetonide
- Fluocinonide
- Halcinonide
- Procinonide
- Triamcinolone
- Triamcinolone acetonide
- Triamcinolone diacetate

Budesonide is a 1:1 mixture of two isomers, the R-and S-isomer. The S-isomer cross-reacts with group D2 corticosteroids such as hydrocortisone-17-butyrate, hydrocortisone-17-aceponate, methylprednisolone aceponate, and prednicarbate. It also cross-reacts with alclometasone dipropionate, belonging to group D1. Therefore, products containing these corticosteroids should also be avoided.

Alternatives	Corticosteroids from group A, C, and D1 except for alclometasone dipropionate (D1).

Examples from group A:
- Cloprednol
- Fludrocortisone acetate
- Hydrocortisone
- Hydrocortisone acetate
- Methylprednisolone
- Prednisolone
- Prednisolone caproate
- Tixocortol pivalate

Examples from group C:
- Betamethasone
- Desoximethasone
- Dexamethasone
- Diflucortolone valerate
- Flumethasone pivalate
- Fluocortolone
- Fluprednidene acetate
- Halomethasone

Examples from group D1:
- Beclomethasone dipropionate
- Betamethasone and its esters, such as valerate and dipropionate
- Clobetasol propionate
- Clobetasone butyrate
- Clobetasone propionate
- Diflorasone diacetate
- Fluticasone propionate
- Mometasone furoate

Tixocortol Pivalate

Designations	**INCI Name.** Tixocortol pivalate.
	CAS No. 55560-96-8.

Test Preparation	• 0.1% pet. (allergen-patch-tape)

Occurrence Tixocortol pivalate is a screening agent for cortico-steroid sensitivity and a marker for group A cortico-steroids, i.e., the hydrocortisone type lacking substitution on the D ring except for a short-chain ester on C_{21} or a thioester on C_{21}. Tixocortol pivalate is present in pharmaceuticals intended for the treatment of rhinitis (as nasal suspension), pharyngitis (as lozenges), ulcerative colitis (as enema and rectal solution), oral, inflammatory conditions (as suspension and powder), and as suspension to be used inside the sinuses.

Products to Avoid Pharmaceuticals containing tixocortol pivalate and potentially cross-reacting corticosteroids should be avoided. This pertains to both topical and systemic pharmaceuticals.

Cross-reactivity Tixocortol pivalate cross-reacts with other cortico-steroids from group A, e.g., hydrocortisone, hydrocortisone acetate, prednisolone, prednisolone caproate, prednisone, fludrocortisone acetate, methylpred-nisolone, and cloprednol. Tixocortol pivalate may also cross-react with the group D2 corticosteroid hydrocortisone-17-butyrate, as this corticosteroid can metabolize to hydrocortisone in the skin.

Alternatives Corticosteroids from group B, C, and D1. Cortico-steroids from group D2 may be tolerated depending on the metabolization in the skin.

Examples from group B:
- Amcinonide
- Budesonide
- Desonide
- Flucloronide
- Flunisolide

- Fluocinolone acetonide
- Fluocinonide
- Halcinonide
- Procinonide
- Triamcinolone
- Triamcinolone acetonide
- Triamcinolone diacetate

Examples from group C:
- Betamethasone
- Desoximethasone
- Dexamethasone
- Diflucortolone valerate
- Flumethasone pivalate
- Fluocortolone
- Flupredniden acetate
- Halomethasone

Examples from group D1:
- Alclometasone dipropionate
- Beclomethasone dipropionate
- Betamethasone dipropionate
- Betamethasone-17-valerate
- Clobetasol propionate
- Clobetasone butyrate
- Clobetasone propionate
- Diflorasone diacetate
- Fluticasone propionate
- Mometasone furoate

Hydrocortisone-17-Butyrate

Designations   **INCI Name.** Hydrocortisone-17-butyrate.
                    CAS No. 13609-67-1.

Test Preparation   - 1.0% ethanol 99.5%v/v (allergen-patch-tape)

Occurrence

Hydrocortisone-17-butyrate is a mid-potent cortico-steroid present in topical pharmaceuticals. It belongs to group D2 (the labile ester corticosteroids), with long-chain ester at C_{17} or C_{17} and C_{21} without C_{16}-methyl substitution and halogenation on the B ring.

Products to Avoid

Topical pharmaceuticals containing hydrocortisone-17-butyrate and potentially cross-reacting cortico-steroids should be avoided.

Cross-reactivity

Hydrocortisone-17-butyrate cross-reacts with other members of group D2 such as methylprednisolone aceponate, hydrocortisone-17-aceponate, hydrocorti-sone-17-buteprate, and prednicarbate. It may cross-react with alclometasone dipropionate from group D1, and it also cross-reacts with the S-isomer of budesonide. Hydrocortisone-17-butyrate can be enzymatically converted to hydrocortisone in the skin, which means that hydrocortisone from group A may not be tolerated. In such cases the patch test to hydrocortisone and/or tixocortol pivalate should be positive.

Alternatives

Corticosteroids from group C and D1 except for alclometasone dipropionate (D1). Corticosteroids from group A and group B with the exception of budesonide (B) may be tolerated depending on skin metabolization.

Examples from group C:
- Betamethasone
- Desoximethasone
- Dexamethasone
- Diflucortolone valerate
- Flumethasone pivalate
- Fluocortolone
- Flupredniden acetate
- Halomethasone

Examples from group D1
- Beclomethasone dipropionate
- Betamethasone dipropionate
- Betamethasone-17-valerate
- Clobetasol propionate
- Clobetasone butyrate
- Clobetasone propionate
- Diflorasone diacetate
- Diflucortolone valerate
- Fluticasone propionate
- Mometasone furoate

References

1. Coopman S, Degreef H, Dooms-Goossens A (1989) Identification of cross-reaction patterns in allergic contact dermatitis from topical corticosteroids. Br J Dermatol 121:27–34
2. Matura M, Goossens A (2000) Contact allergy to corticosteroids. Allergy 55:698–704
3. Isaksson M, Brandão FM, Bruze M, Goossens A (2000) Recommendation to include budesonide and tixocortol pivalate in the European standard series. Contact Dermatitis 43:41–42
4. Isaksson M, Andersen KE, Brandão FM et al. (2000) Patch testing with corticosteroid mixes in Europe. A multicentre study of the EECDRG. Contact Dermatitis 42:27–35
5. Sommer S, Wilkinson SM, English JSC et al. (2002) Type-IV hypersensitivity to betamethasone valerate and clobetasol propionate: results of a multicentre study. Br J Dermatol 147:266–269
6. Isaksson M, Bruze M (2002) Allergic contact dermatitis in response to budesonide reactivated by inhalation of the allergen. J Am Acad Dermatol 46:880–885
7. Bircher AJ, Bigliardi P, Zaugg T, Mäkinen-Kiljunen S (2000) Delayed generalized allergic reactions to corticosteroids. Dermatology 200:349–351

Additional Topical Remedies

Benzocaine

Stefania Seidenari

Designations	**INCI Name.** Benzocaine. **Synonyms.** Ethyl aminobenzoate; anesthesin; anesthone; parathesin. **CAS No.** 94-09-7.
Test Preparation	• 5% pet. (allergen-patch-tape)
Occurrence	Benzocaine is a local and topical anesthetic used in a great number of products, including burn and sunburn remedies, external analgesics, creams for treatment of poison ivy and athlete's foot, suppositories, sore throat sprays/lozenges, antitussives, hemorrhoidal creams, insect-bite remedies, appetite suppressants, astringents, corn, callus, and wart remedies, preparations for toothache, teething, canker sore and denture irritation. It is applied in every orifice of the body (ear, mouth, vagina, and rectum) and in intertriginous areas, which favors sensitization. As a result of such wide use, benzocaine has become a common cause of contact allergy, mainly in countries such as the United States, where it is present in many over-the-counter preparations. The incidence of contact sensitivity to benzocaine in eczema patients is reported to range from 0.8% to 1.5%, according to the level of its use in the country.
Cross-reactivity	Benzocaine is a para-aminoazobenzoic acid (PABA) derivative and cross-reacts with local ester anesthet-

ics and with other para-amino compounds. The parabens are parahydroxy compounds that do not appear to cross-react with para-amino compounds.

Products to Avoid

Benzocaine-sensitive subjects should not use ester anesthetics, both topical and injectable, i.e.:
- Tetracaine
- Procaine
- Cocaine
- Propoxycaine
- Meprylcaine
- Buthetamine
- Metabuthetamine

They should also avoid all products containing:
- Procainamide
- PABA and glyceryl PABA (sunscreens)
- PPD
- Azoaniline dyes
- Hydrochlorothiazide
- Sulfonamides
- Sulfonylureas
- Aminosalicylic acid

Alternatives

Local amide anesthetics, i.e.: lidocaine, mepivacaine, prilocaine, pramocaine, pyrrocaine, and dibucaine.

References

1. Fischer AA (1986) Contact dermatitis, 3rd edn. Lea and Febiger, Philadelphia, pp 220–223
2. Kanerva L (2001) Skin diseases from dental materials. In: Rycroft RJG, Mennè T, Frosch PJ, Lepoittevin JP (eds) Textbook of contact dermatitis, 3rd edn. Springer, Berlin Heidelberg New York, pp 862–863

Cetylstearyl Alcohol

MATTI HANNUKSELA

INCI Name. Cetearyl alcohol.
Synonyms. Cetostearol; Lanette O.
CAS No. 8005-44-5.

Test Preparation

• 20% pet. (allergen-patch-tape)

Occurrence

Cetylstearyl alcohol (CSA) is a popular emulsifier in cream bases. It contains both cetyl (C_{16}) and stearyl (C_{18}) alcohols. The cosmetic grade of CSA contains 3–4% other alcohols, the composition of which are not fully known. In a study of cetyl alcohol allergy, the test substance was found to contain, in addition to the main component, stearyl (C_{18}), myristyl (C_{14}), and lauryl (C_{12}) alcohols [1]. In another study, chromatographic analysis of commercial Lanette 16 revealed 92.1% cetyl alcohol, 3.3% stearyl alcohol, while the rest contained mainly C_8–C_{14} alcohols [2]. Lanette N, another popular emulsifier, contains 80–90% Lanette O and 10–20% sodium cetylstearyl sulfate. CSA is usually patch tested at 20% in petrolatum. Cetyl alcohol is said to be more irritant than stearyl alcohol [3], while Lanette N has been claimed to be nonirritant [4]. When tested separately, cetyl alcohol can be tested at 5% and stearyl alcohol at 30% in petrolatum [3].

CSA and other higher fatty alcohols produce positive (allergic) patch-test reactions usually in 0.5–1.0% of patients with eczematous dermatitis [2, 5, 6] while

the number of reactors is much higher, up to 30%, in
leg ulcer patients [7, 8, 9]. Chemically pure alcohols
have been found to produce positive patch-test reactions only occasionally. The number of irritant
reactions is not usually given. We found irritant responses to Lanette N in 4 of 1,206 (0.4%) dermatitis
patients [5].

The relevance of a positive patch-test reaction re-
mains to be further studied using the repeated open
application test (ROAT) or some other usage test.
Fourteen of sixteen patients with + or ++ patch-test
reaction to 20% Lanette N showed positive response
in the ROAT with the test substance. The corresponding number for 30% Lanette 16 was two of three
patients [2, 6]. In a study by Tosti [6], the clinical relevance of a positive patch-test reaction to 20% CSA
was definitely established in three of six patients. A
series of 11 leg ulcer patients with + to ++ patch-test
reactions to 20% CSA were retested with 20% CSA,
5% cetyl alcohol, and 30% stearyl alcohol [3]. Only
one patient reacted to CSA and stearyl alcohol and
one patient to stearyl alcohol only. The results of a
ROAT with a cream containing 8% CSA were negative in all patients.

In summary, CSA and other higher fatty alcohols are
recommended to be patch tested in vehicle series.
Positive reactions should be interpreted with caution,
especially in leg ulcer patients. The clinical relevance
of positive reactions should be confirmed with the
ROAT or other usage tests.

References

1. Komamura H, Doi T, Inui S, Yoshikawa K (1997) A case of
   contact dermatitis due to impurities of cetyl alcohol.
   Contact Dermatitis 36:44–46
2. Hannuksela M, Salo H (1986) The repeated open application
   test (ROAT). Contact Dermatitis 14:221–227
3. Werth JM von det, English JSC, Dalziel KL (1998) Loss
   of patch test positivity to cetylstearyl alcohol. Contact
   Dermatitis 38:109–110

4. Bandmann H-J, Dohn W (1967) Die Epikutantestung.
   Bergman, Munich
5. Hannuksela M, Kousa M, Pirilä V (1976) Contact sensitivity
   to emulsifiers. Contact Dermatitis 2:201–204
6. Tosti A, Guerra L, Morelli R, Bardazzi F (1990) Prevalence
   and sources of sensitization to emulsifiers: a clinical study.
   Contact Dermatitis 23:68–72
7. Blondeel A, Oleffe J, Achten G (1978) Contact allergy in 330
   dermatological patients. Contact Dermatitis 4:270–276
8. Bandmann H-J, Keilig W (1980) Lanett O – another test substance for lower leg series. Contact Dermatitis 6:227–228
9. Keilig W (1983) Kontaktallergie auf Cetylstearylalkohol
   (Lanette O) als therapeutische Problem bei Stauungs-
   dermatitis und Ulcus cruris. Derm Beruf Umwelt 31:50–54

Clioquinol

JEAN-MARIE LACHAPELLE

Designations

INCI Name. Clioquinol.
Synonyms. Chinoform; chloroiodoquine; iodochlorhydroxyquin; iodochlorhydroxyquinoleine; 5-chloro-7-iodoquinolin-8-ol; Vioform.
CAS No. 130-26-7.

Test Preparations

- Clioquinol 5% pet. (allergen-patch-tape)
  Due to stability problems, clioquinol 5% pet. has replaced the quinoline mix in the standard series. The quinoline mix (clioquinol 3% pet. + chlorquinaldol 3% pet.) is still used in the USA
- Quinoline mix (equal parts of clioquinol and chlorquinaldol) in hydroxypropylcellulose. Total concentration, 190 µg/cm^2 (TRUE-test system)
  Clioquinol is a synthetic anti-infective (antibacterial and, to a lesser extent, antifungal) agent. Clioquinol (and chlorquinaldol) are quinoline derivates [1].

Occurrence

Clioquinol has been used widely as a topical anti-infective (antibacterial and antifungal) agent (Vioform, topical dermatological formulations, e.g., Vioform and zinc paste, in the UK). Its use has decreased substantially since the advent of new topical antibiotics and/or antifungals. Clioquinol has also been used systemically to treat various infections, including amebiasis. Chlorquinaldol (5,6-dichloro-2-methyl-quinolin-8-ol), a closely related quinoline derivate, has also been used systemically for the same purpose

(Sterosan, Steroxin). Both are prescribed less and less, and are even suppressed in some countries.

Cross-reactions between clioquinol and chlorquinaldol are not common. When administered systemically in patients with allergic contact dermatitis to clioquinol, both can provoke systemic contact dermatitis. This could be true also for other systemically administered quinolones such as norfloxacin, ofloxacin, and ciprofloxacin, which are largely used for their widespectrum antibacterial properties [2].

Independent of this, quinolones are responsible for several variants of drug eruptions. These skin reactions have no link with allergic contact dermatitis. They can occur in patients with no contact allergy to clioquinol, and, due to their unpredictability, no preventive measures can be achieved [3].

Chemically related substances include chlorquinaldol, diiodohydroxyquin, chlorhydroxyquinoline, quinolones (norfloxacin, ofloxacin, ciprofloxacin, etc.).

Products to Avoid

Patients who are allergic to clioquinol should inform all of their health care providers of their allergy [4]. Clioquinol has to be avoided topically and/or systemically. A similar prevention is applied to the oral administration of chlorquinaldol and of recent quinolones (norfloxacin, ofloxacin, ciprofloxacin, etc), bearing in mind the nonnegligible risk of systemic contact dermatitis.

References

1. Andersen KE, White IR, Goossens A (2001) Allergens of the standard series. In: Rycroft RJG, Menné T, Frosch PJ, Lepoittevin JP (eds) Textbook of contact dermatitis 3rd edn, chap 31. Springer, Berlin Heidelberg New York, pp 629–630
2. Silvestre JF, Alonso R, Moragon M, Ramon R, Botella R (1998) Systemic contact dermatitis due to norfoxacin with a positive patch test to quinoline mix. Contact Dermatitis 39:83
3. Litt Z (2001) Drug eruption reference manual. Parthenon, New York, p 245
4. Marks JG, Elsner P, Leo VA de (2002) Contact and occupational dermatology, 3rd edn. Mosby, St Louis, pp 130–132

Ethylenediamine Dihydrochloride

Susanne Freeman

Designations	**INCI Name.** Ethylenediamine dihydrochloride. **CAS No.** 333-18-6.
Test Preparations	• 1.0% pet. (allergen-patch-tape) • 50 µg/cm² (TRUE-test system) Ethylenediamine is now a rare sensitizer and may be removed from the standard series.
Occurrence	Ethylenediamine dihydrochloride is found in floor-polish remover, epoxy hardener, and coolant oil. In industry, it is used in rubber, dyes, insecticides, and synthetic waxes. Previously (but no longer) ethylenediamine dihydrochloride was present as a stabilizer in Mycolog, Tri-adcortyl, and Kenacomb creams.
Products to Avoid	Avoid aminophylline (contains ethylenediamine) and systemic drugs that can cross-react (v.i.).
Cross-reactivity	Antihistamines, e.g., hydroxyzine hydrochloride, piperazine, cyclizine.
Reference	1. Andersen KE, White I R, Goossens A (2001) Allergens from the standard series. In: Rycroft RJG, Menne T, Frosch PJ, Lepoittevin J-P (eds) Textbook of contact dermatitis. Springer, Berlin Heidelberg New York, pp 657–658

Neomycin Sulfate

AN GOOSSENS

Designations	**INCI Name.** Neomycin sulfate. **CAS No.** 1404-04-2.
Test Preparations	• 20% pet. (allergen-patch-tape) • 230 µg/cm² (TRUE-test system)
Occurrence	Neomycin, an aminoglycoside antibiotic derived from *Streptomyces fradiae*, is a mixture of two isomers, neomycin B (78–88%) and neomycin C (10–16%) with neomycin A (neamin). It is used in many medications for external use such as creams, powders, ointments, and ear, nose, and eye drops, for the treatment of infections. Sensitization occurs generally by application to leg ulcers. Neomycin sulfate is also used as an antibiotic for internal use (systemic administration can cause generalized eczematous reactions in sensitized persons). It is also used in veterinary medicine for internal preparations. Neomycin sulfate is used in vaccines. It is also added to pet food and chicken feed (now forbidden in the EC).

Cross-reactions   Neomycin sulfate may cross-react with other amino-
                         glycosides such as:
                         - Amitracin
                         - Arbekacin
                         - Butirosin
                         - Dibekacin
                         - Framycetin
                         - Gentamycin
                         - Isepamicin
                         - Kanamycin
                         - Netilmicin
                         - Paromomycin
                         - Ribostamycin
                         - Sisomycin
                         - Streptomycin
                         - Tobramycin

References   1. Parfitt K (ed) (1999) Martindale. The complete drug refer-
                            ence, 32nd edn. Pharmaceutical, London, pp 229–231
                         2. Andersen K, White IR, Goossens A (2001) Allergens from
                            the standard series, chap 31, 3rd edn. In: Rycroft RJG,
                            Menné T, Frosh PJ, Lepoittevin JP (eds) Textbook of contact
                            dermatitis. Springer, Berlin Heidelberg New York, pp 627–628

Propylene Glycol

MAHBUB M.U. CHOWDHURY, HOWARD I. MAIBACH

Designations

INCI Name. Propylene glycol.
Synonyms. At least 13 reported.
CAS No. 57-55-6.

Test Preparation

- 5% pet.; 20% aq. (allergen-patch-tape)
  Varies, not finally stated.

Occurrence

Propylene glycol is an excellent vehicle and solvent for dermatological and nondermatological products. It has antimicrobial and antifungal properties, particularly above 25% concentration. Propylene glycol has substituted glycerin in many products due to increased lipid solubility, and hence better permeation of the stratum corneum, and is also less expensive. It is used in topical agents, including corticosteroid creams and ointments, cosmetics, ear and eye treatments, and also personal hygiene products such as shampoos, antiperspirants, and shaving creams. It is also present in K-Y jelly and gels used for electrocardiography and transcutaneous electrical nerve stimulator units. Industrial uses include: tobacco humectant, brake-fluid component, antifreeze, and solvent and preservative in the food industry. Propylene glycol can also be found in some oral antibiotics and parenteral therapies such as diazepam, phenytoin and lorazepam, with a concentration of up to 40%.

Positive Patch Test   A combination of tests is required to confirm allergic contact dermatitis to propylene glycol. Repeat patch-testing should be performed in all patients who have tested positive after some weeks. Undiluted, 50% and 10% propylene glycol can all be a skin irritant, especially under occlusion. In atopics, propylene glycol concentrations as low as 5% can cause irritation. Irritant reactions are more common in winter, and this is possibly related to increased transepidermal water loss due to the hygroscopic nature of propylene glycol. Irritation and sensitization patch-test studies in combination with the provocative use test (PUT) indicate that propylene glycol is at least a minimal irritant.

Concentrations above 10% may be incorrectly interpreted as allergic reactions and testing at concentrations lower than 10% may miss true positive reactions. Most authors recommend a concentration of between 1% and 10%; however, repeated open application tests (ROAT) have concluded that a patch-test concentration of between 10% and 30% propylene glycol may be desirable. Some cases have been missed with concentrations below 50% propylene glycol.

An algorithm has been suggested for the diagnosis of propylene glycol dermatitis. Any positive propylene glycol patch test requires a combination of tests for an objective assessment. This includes serial dilutions, ROAT/PUT, and if necessary oral challenge tests prior to long-term prohibition and avoidance of propylene glycol.

Cross-reactivity   Not reported.

References

1. Niklasson BJ (2000) List of patch test allergens. In: Kanerva L, Elsner P, Wahlberg JE, Maibach HI (eds) Handbook of occupational dermatology. Springer, Berlin Heidelberg New York, p 1232
2. Funk JO, Maibach HI (1994) Propylene glycol dermatitis: re-evaluation of an old problem. Contact Dermatitis 31: 236–241
3. Hannuksela M, Pirilä V, Salo OP (1975) Skin reactions to propylene glycol. Contact Dermatitis 1:112–116
4. Hannuksela M, Forstom L (1978) Reactions to peroral propylene glycol. Contact Dermatitis 4:41–45
5. Frosch PJ, Pekar U, Enzmann H (1990) Contact allergy to propylene glycol: do we use the appropriate test concentration? Dermatol Clin 8:111–113
6. Wahlberg JE (1994) Propylene glycol: search for a proper and non-irritant patch test preparation. Am J Contact Dermatitis 5:156–159

Wool Alcohols

AN GOOSSENS

Designations	**INCI Name.** Lanolin alcohol.
	Synonyms. Wool wax alcohol; lanolin (EU).
	CAS No. 8027-33-6.
Test Preparations	• 30% pet. (allergen-patch-tape)
	• 1,000 µg/cm² (TRUE-test system)
Occurrence	Wool alcohols are a complex mixture of organic alcohols obtained from the hydrolysis of lanolin, a natural product from sheep fleece. Derivatives include: lanolin acid, oil, and wax; lanolin esters; alkoxylated lanolin carboxy acids and lanolin alcohols; hydrogenated derivatives; and sterols.

Wool alcohols are used as binders, emulsion stabilizers, hair-conditioning agents, and viscosity-increasing agents. Wool alcohols are widely used in:

- Topical pharmaceutical products (including adhesive plasters and self-adhesive dressings)
- Cosmetics (skin-care and hair preparations, make up, suntan products, cleansing products, shaving products)

Wool alcohols are also used in:
- Printing inks
- Polishes
- Anticorrosives
- Paper constituents
- Materials for sealing metals

- Cooling fluids for metals
- Impregnation agents for textiles and leatherwear
- Ski wax
- Insulation for wiring

Chemically related substances include lanolin derivatives, wool fat, and Eucerin.

Products to Avoid   All products containing lanolin alcohols or related materials. The most important cause of contact allergy to these substances consists of locally applied pharmaceuticals, for example, in the treatment of leg ulcers or stasis dermatitis.

References

1. Andersen K, White IR, Goossens A (2001) Allergens from the standard series. In: Rycroft RJG, Menné T, Frosh PJ, Lepoittevin JP (eds). Textbook of contact dermatitis, chap 31, 3rd edn. Springer, Berlin Heidelberg New York, pp 630–631
2. Wenninger JA, Canterbery RC, McEwen GN (eds) (1999) International cosmetic ingredient dictionary and handbook. Cosmetic, Toiletry and Fragrance Association, Washington DC, pp 756–766

Plants

Colophony

GUNILLA FÄRM

Designations

INCI Name. Colophonium.
Synonyms. Rosin; disproportionated rosin; gum rosin; wood rosin; pine rosin; rosin solder flux fume.
CAS No. 8050-09-7.

Test Preparations

- 20% pet. (allergen-patch-tape)
- 1,200 µg/cm² (TRUE-test system)

Occurrence

Colophony is a naturally occurring material obtained from different species of coniferous tree. Much of the world production of colophony is used in the paper industry to increase the water resistance of paper. Colophony has a very good adhesive property and is therefore used in many sticky products. You will find colophony in the following products: wood and gum from pine trees; adhesives, glues, and tapes, including plaster and adhesive bandages; printing ink; some paints and lacquers; and polishes. Colophony is also commonly found in soldering fluxes. Cosmetics may contain colophony, particularly mascara, but also bindi (used by Asian women) and depilatory waxes. Some dental material contains colophony and it may be found in some chewing gum. Dancers' and string-players' rosin consists of colophony.

Products to Avoid

Be careful to read the label of products made for skin care or cosmetic purposes to be sure they do not contain colophony (rosin). In the European Union all products containing 1% colophony or more have to be labeled with an allergy warning. Tell your dentist and your doctor to avoid colophony-containing materials. Try to avoid skin contact with glues, adhesives, and tapes, as well as with paints, lacquers, and cooling fluids. Always check the labeling. Ordinary paper work generally does not cause contact dermatitis.

Cross-reactivity

Colophony is often modified chemically. The allergenicity might then change. Sometimes, however, there is enough unmodified colophony left in the new product to cause dermatitis. The modified colophony might have a trade name which does not contain "colophony" or "rosin" (among others, Staybelite, Hercolyne, Pentalyn, Abitol), which makes it difficult for the consumer to identify.

Alternatives

There are several colophony-free adhesive tapes. Many mascaras do not contain colophony.

References

1. Karlberg A-T (1988) Contact allergy to colophony. Chemical identifications of allergens, sensitization experiments and clinical experiences. Acta Derm Venereol (Stockh) (Suppl) 139:1–43
2. Färm G (1998) Contact allergy to colophony. Clinical and experimental studies with emphasis on clinical relevance. Acta Derm Venereol (Stockh) (Suppl) 201:1–42

Primin

MONICA HINDSÉN

Designations	**Synonym.** 2-Methoxy-6-pentyl-1,4-benzoquinone.
Test Preparation	• 0.01% pet. (allergen-patch-tape)
Occurrence	Primin is known to be present only in the plant *Primula obconica*.
Products to Avoid	Individuals with primin allergy should avoid handling *Primula obconica* plants and they should not keep *Primula obconica* plants in rooms where they work or live, to avoid airborne contact dermatitis.
Cross-reactivity	Cross-reactivity has been suggested to miconidin (2-methoxy-6-pentyl-1,4-dihydroxybenzene), another *Primula obconica* allergen.

References

1. Fregert S, Hjort N (1977) The primula allergen primin. Contact Dermatitis 3:172–174
2. Christensen LP, Larsen E (2000) Direct emission of the allergen primin from intact *Primula obconica* plants. Contact Dermatitis 42:149–153

Sesquiterpene Lactone Mix

EVY PAULSEN, KLAUS E. ANDERSEN

The sesquiterpene lactone mix (SL mix) consists of 3 allergens: alantolactone, costunolide, dehydrocostus lactone.

Alantolactone

Designations   **INCI Name.** Alantolactone.
Synonyms. Alant camphor; elecampane camphor; inula camphor; Eupatal.
CAS No. 546-43-0.

Costunolide

Designations   **INCI Name.** Costunolide.
CAS No. 553-21-9.

Dehydrocostus lactone

Designations   **INCI Name.** Dehydrocostus lactone.
CAS No. 477-43-0.

Test Preparation   • 0.1% pet. (allergen-patch-tape)

Occurrence A positive patch-test reaction to the sesquiterpene
lactone (SL) mix suggests that the patient is allergic
to plants containing SL allergens. There are more
than 1,600 SLs in nature, and the distribution of
these allergens is only partly clarified. The largest
SL-containing plant family, however, is the daisy
family (Compositae, Asteraceae), but SLs may also
be found in other families. Allergic contact eczema
caused by plants of the Compositae family
(Compositae dermatitis) is well known in Europe,
the USA, India, and Australia. The symptoms may
be eczema of hands and/or face or more widespread
dermatitis that typically occurs or worsens in
summer.

The Compositae family is comprised of: weeds such
as yarrow (*Achillea millefolium*), tansy (*Tanacetum
vulgare*), chamomile (*Chamomilla recutita*), dande-
lion (*Taraxacum officinale*), short ragweed (*Ambrosia
artemisiifolia*), and capeweed (*Arctotheca calendu-
lacea*); cultivated ornamental plants such as florists'
chrysanthemums (*Dendranthema*), sunflower
(*Helianthus annuus*), marguerite (*Argyranthemum
frutescens*), and marigold (*Calendula officinalis*);
and vegetables/spices such as lettuce (*Lactuca sativa*),
chicory (*Cichorium intybus*), endive (*Cichorium
endivia*), globe artichoke (*Cynara scolymus*), viper's
grass (*Scorzonera hispanica*), Jerusalem artichoke
(*Helianthus tuberosus*), salsify (*Tragopogon porri-
folius*), and estragon (*Artemisia dracunculus*) [1, 2, 3].

Plants and Products Since the allergens are widely distributed in the
to Avoid Compositae family, it would be theoretically best,
but hardly practically possible, to avoid contact with
all species of this family. Depending on the degree
of sensitivity, it may be sufficient to remove a few
offending species from the house and/or garden in
case of weak, relevant patch-test reactions, or remove
all Compositae species in case of strongly positive

reactions. Although the use of gloves is recommended, it may not be sufficient to avoid contact with
allergens during gardening or cleansing/handling
of vegetables. Although many SL-sensitive patients
may enjoy salads with lettuce or other Compositae
vegetables without problems, ingestion of edible
Compositae plants or herbal teas in some cases may
worsen the eczema within hours or days and even induce symptoms of the mucous membranes. Furthermore, many Compositae plants are used in herbal
medicine (e.g. arnica and chamomile) and cosmetics
(e.g., *Calendula*); avoid such over-the-counter products and "homemade" remedies such as chamomile
tea compresses [2].

Examples of specific plants that contain allergen(s)
of the SL mix:
- Alantolactone: In the garden plants elecampane
  (*Inula helenium*), *Inula grandis*, and other *Inula*
  species. The SL isoalantolactone that cross-reacts
  with alantolactone is found in great yellow ox-eye
  (*Telekia speciosa*).
- Costunolide: In garden plants such as elecampane
  (*Inula helenium*), annual garden cosmeas (*Cosmos
  sulphureus* and an unidentified *Cosmos* cultivar,
  although it is probably not the major allergen), in
  bay leaf (*Laurus nobilis*), and in the liverwort
  Frullania tamarisci.
- Dehydrocostus lactone: In the ornamental garden
  plants *Stokesia laevis* and *Vernonia hirsuta*.

Cross-reactivity

Besides cross-reactivity within the daisy family, there
are cross-reacting species within other plant families
such as, e.g., Magnoliaceae (including *Magnolia*
species), Lauraceae (including bay leaf), Apiaceae
(umbelliferous plants), and Frullaniaceae and other
liverwort families. Persons with Compositae allergy
should not get into direct contact with leaves or

flowers of, e.g., *Magnolia stellata* or *Magnolia grandiflora*, and likewise avoid contact with liverwort growing on trees (including chopped firewoood with bark). Ingestion of food spiced with bay leaf may cause flares of eczema.

References

1. Guin JD (1989) Sesquiterpene-lactone dermatitis. Immunol Allergy Clin North Am 9:447–461
2. Lovell CR (1993) Plants and the skin. Blackwell Scientific Publications, Oxford
3. Paulsen E (1992) Compositae dermatitis: a survey. Contact Dermatitis 26:76–86

Urushiol

Jere D. Guin

Designations	**INCI Name.** Urushiol. **Sources.** Poison ivy (*Toxicodendron radicans*); Eastern poison oak (*T. toxicarium*); poison sumac (*T. vernix*); Japanese lacquer tree (*T. verniciflua*). **CAS No.** 492-89-7.
Test Preparation	Not normally tested because of tendency to cause sensitization or to heighten preexisting sensitivity. Most testing done as research method, often with serial dilution. Japanese lacquer, if available, is a suitable test mate- rial for poison ivy, oak, and sumac. It may be less specific for some other members of the Anacar- diaceae. Oleoresin from the plant can also be used if properly diluted. The test is usually open as 0.05–2.5 µg in acetone. Higher concentrations should be avoided.
Occurrence	Urushiol is found in poison ivy, oak, and sumac, and in the Japanese lacquer tree.
Cross-reactivity	Cross-reactivity with *Ginkgo biloba* seed, certain Proteaceae (*Grevillea robusta*, etc.), and many other toxicodendrons, as well as the (toxic) Anacardiaceae, e.g.: • *Anacardium* • *Comocladia* • *Gluta*

- *Holigarna*
- *Lannea*
- *Lithraea*
- *Mangifera*
- *Mauria*
- *Melanochyla*
- *Metopium*
- *Nothopegia* (possibly)
- *Pentaspadon*
- *Pseudosmodingium*
- *Smodingium*
- *Semecarpus*

and perhaps *Swintonia*.

References

1. Epstein WL, Byers VS, Frankart W (1982) Induction of antigen-specific hyposensitization to poison oak in sensitized adults. Arch Dermatol 118:630–633
2. Guin JD, Beaman JH, Baer H (1999) Toxic Anacardiaceae. In: Avalos J, Maibach HI (eds) Dermatologic botany. CRC Press, Boca Raton, pp 85–142

Miscellaneous

Epoxy Resin

RIITTA JOLANKI, KRISTIINA ALANKO

Designations

INCI Name. Epoxy resin.
Synonyms. Diglycidyl ether of bisphenol A epoxy resin; DGEBA epoxy resin; epichlorohydrin/bisphenol A epoxy resin.
CAS No. 25068-38-6.

Test Preparations

- 1% pet. (allergen-patch-tape)
- 50 µg/cm² TRUE-test system

Occurrence

Epoxy resins are synthetic resins used to make plastics and adhesives. The resins are noted for their versatility, but their relatively high cost has limited their use. Up to 95% of epoxy resins used worldwide are reaction products of epichlorohydrin (CAS no. 106-89-8) and bisphenol A [CAS no. 80-05-7; synonym, 2,2-bis(4-hydroxyphenyl)propane]. Epichlorohydrin/bisphenol A epoxy resins, usually called DGEBA-type epoxy resins, are generally mixtures of monomers, diglycidyl-ether-of-bisphenol-A (DGEBA) molecules with a molecular weight (MW) of 340, and oligomer molecules with a higher MW. The DGEBA has the highest sensitizing capacity. Liquid epoxy resins (mean MW of 350–400) contain even more than 90% DGEBA. Even solid resins (mean MW of over 900) may contain more than 15% DGEBA. The epoxy resin patch-test substance is made of the liquid DGEBA-type epoxy resin. Non-DGEBA epoxy resins possess special properties that have made them competitive with DGEBA resins for certain applications. Non-DGEBA epoxy resins such as brominated epoxy resins and epoxy resins based on diglycidyl ether of bisphenol F (DGEBF) may also contain DGEBA epoxy resin.

Epoxy resins are normally used in what is called an epoxy-resin system. The system usually consists of two components, a resin component and a curing agent (hardener). After the two epoxy components are mixed, there is a working time (pot life) during which the epoxy can be applied or used. In a few minutes or hours, a chemical reaction occurs between the components, generating heat and causing hardening of the mixture at either an ambient or an elevated temperature. At the end of the pot life, the mixture may become dangerously hot, which helps volatile components evaporate into the air. One-component epoxy products also exist; they contain curing agents which are inactive at storage temperatures, but which initiate a curing process when heated. The term ‹epoxy resin› may refer to the resins in both the uncured and the cured state. Once epoxy resin becomes hardened, its sensitizing capacity is markedly reduced, but cured resins can still contain uncured sensitizing molecules and can thus induce sensitization. Apart from resin molecules, epoxy products also contain other sensitizing chemicals; the most prominent are reactive diluents and curing agents. Other additives include fillers, tar, colorants, UV-light absorbers, flame-retardants, solvents, reinforcements, non-epoxy resins, and plasticizers.

Epoxy resins are commonly used in everyday life as adhesives (Table 1). They form tough bonds on metal and many other surfaces such as plastics, rubber, wood, glass, and ceramics. The selection of epoxy adhesives ranges from those used as two-package, ambient-cure, general adhesives in domestic applications to high-performance, one-component sheet adhesives for aircraft assembly.

The high resistance of epoxy resins to chemicals and their hardness, outstanding adhesion, and durability properties have made them valuable as two-component paints, lacquers, and other protective coatings (Table 1). Because of their high electrical resistance, epoxy resins are used in insulation resins and tapes (manufacture of condensers and electrical motors) or to encapsulate electrical and electronic components (assembly of electrical and electronic devices). The resins are used as casting resin and in the manufacture of glass fibers as sizing agents, and in floor-

Table 1. Exposing situations or products containing epoxy resin

Two-component adhesives

Two-component paints, lacquers, and other coatings

- Anticorrosion protection for metals (e.g., ocean liners, and oil-drilling platforms)
- Waterproof protection for concrete
- Chemical-resistant protection for floors and walls

Electrical insulation and encapsulation

Casting resin

Glass-fiber manufacture

Concrete injection, flooring, and stonework

Epoxy composite manufacture

- Pipes and vessels
- Sporting goods (tennis racquets, skis, ski poles, and fishing rods)
- Automotive, boat-building, and aircraft industries
- Military and aerospace applications
- Electrical applications (e.g., electronic circuit boards)

Embedding resin for electron microscopy, microscopy immersion oil

Lamination resin, prepreg-laminates

Powder epoxy and epoxy-polyester paints

Nail coatings

ing materials and stonework. They are also used as injection resins to repair cracks in concrete, and in the manufacture of composite products (Table 1). Epoxy resins may also be used in the preparation of samples for electron microscopy. An unexpected recent source of epoxy resin is microscopy immersion oil. Lamination resins and even nail polishes may contain epoxy resin. One-component products are used mainly in the electrical industry and as powder paints, one-pack glues, and prepreg laminates.

Cross-reactivity   DGEBA epoxy resins do not cause cross allergy with other epoxy compounds such as reactive diluents. Cross-reactivity is possible with epoxy dimethacrylates such as BIS-GMA, used in dental composite materials.

Alternatives   The use of less-sensitizing products may reduce the possibility of developing allergy to epoxy resin, as resins with high MW do not sensitize readily. The use of one-bag epoxy products, which mix in the package, may reduce the possibility of skin contact. An automatic process, as such, does not guarantee protection against skin exposure, for example, during maintenance, repair, or sampling.

Protection. Gloves made of laminated, multilayered plastic (4H-glove), developed especially for the handling of epoxy resin products give the best protection. The use of any type of gloves, however, seems to reduce the exposure to epoxy resin compounds and helps to protect against the risk of sensitization, although the use of protective gloves may, in some individual cases, even promote contact allergens to come into contact with the skin. Unhealthy skin, including even small cuts and abrasions, should be protected from epoxy-compound exposure because of increased skin penetration.

Because airborne exposure to epoxy resin components is also possible, the airways should also be
protected from exposure to epoxy compounds,
because, apart from skin sensitizers, these compounds can be considered potential causes of rhinitis
and asthma.

References

1. Björkner B (2001) Plastic materials. In: Rycroft RJG,
   Menné T, Frosch PJ, Lepoittevin J-P (eds) Textbook of
   contact dermatitis. Springer, Berlin Heidelberg New York,
   pp 783–824
2. Jolanki R, Kanerva L, Estlander T (2000) Epoxy resins.
   In: Kanerva L, Elsner P, Wahlberg JE, Maibach HI (eds)
   Handbook of occupational dermatology. Springer, Berlin
   Heidelberg New York, pp 570–590

para-Phenylenediamine Free Base

Stefania Seidenari

Designations	**INCI Name.** PPD, 4-phenylenediamine. **CAS No.** 105-50-3.
Test Preparations	• 1% pet. (allergen-patch-tape) in a dark bottle • 90 µg/cm² (TRUE-test system)
Occurrence	PPD is a primary intermediate in permanent hair dyes and fur dyes. It is a colorless compound that is oxidized by hydrogen peroxide and then polymerized by a coupling agent to produce a color. Most cases of sensitization to PPD are caused by contact with hair dyes, both in the clients and in the hairdressers. Once the hair is dyed and polymerized, it is nonsensitizing; however, cases of people reacting to another person's dyed hair have been reported, when the dyeing has not been carried out properly and the unoxidized product remains on the hair. PPD is also used in photographic developing, lithography, photocopying, X-ray fluids, greases, oils, gasoline, and as antioxidant/accelerator in the rubber and plastic industry. It can be found as a cause of contact dermatitis in violinists due to chin-rest stains and in water and milk testers because of PPD content in reagents. PPD is also employed as a skin paint, added to henna mixtures for temporary tattoos. The frequency of PPD allergy ranges from 2.8% to 7.1%, with considerable geographical variations.

Cross-reactivity

Cross-reactions may occur to other para-amino compounds. Therefore PPD-sensitive subjects should be warned about the use of local anesthetics, sulfonamides, anthraquinone, PABA sunscreens, parabens, diaminodiphenylmethane, antihistamines, the rubber antioxidant 4-isopropylaminodiphenylamine, and aniline and azo dyes. Among azo dyes, cosensitizations to PPD are more frequently observed in Disperse Orange 3-, PAAB-, and PDAAB-sensitive patients than in Disperse Blue 106/124-sensitive patients. Some food additives (i.e., Citrus Red 2 and Sunset Yellow) also have formulas suggesting possible cross-reactions to PPD. However, data about cross-sensitization rates are lacking for most haptens, and each patient has to be considered individually.

PPD cross-reacts to other related hair dyes such as *p*-toluendiamine; *p*-aminodiphenylamine; 2,4-daminoanisole; and *o*-aminophenol. Therefore patients sensitized to PPD should use alternative hair dyes, i.e., henna or new-generation hair dyes.

References

1. Lepoittevin JP, Le Coz C (2000) Dictionary of occupational allergens. In: Kanerva L, Elsner P, Wahlberg JE, Maibach HI (eds) Handbook of occupational dermatology. Springer, Berlin Heidelberg New York, p 1165
2. Andersen K (2001) Allergens from the standard series. In: Rycroft RJG, Mennè T, Frosch PJ, Lepoittevin JP (eds) Textbook of contact dermatitis, 3rd edn. Springer, Berlin Heidelberg New York, pp 640–642
3. Maibach HI, Engasser PG (1986) Dermatitis due to cosmetics. In: Fischer AA (ed) Contact dermatitis, 3rd edn. Lea and Febiger, Philadelphia, pp 380–382
4. Fautz R, Fuchs A, Walle H van der, Henny V, Smits L (2002) Hair dye-sensitized hairdressers: the cross-reaction pattern with new generation hair dyes. Contact Dermatitis 46:319–324

p-Tertiary-Butylphenol Formaldehyde Resin

CHEE LEOK GOH

Designations

Synonyms. Paratertiary butylphenol formaldehyde resin; PTBP formaldehyde; PTBP-F-R; butylphen; 4(1,1-dimethylethyl)phenol.

Test Preparations

- 1% pet. (allergen-patch-tape)
- 45 µg/cm² (TRUE-test system)

Patients should be tested for PTBP-FR and should also be tested for relevant associated chemicals such as PTBP, HCHO, and phenol formaldehyde resin (P-FR).

Occurrence

p-Tertiary-butylphenol formaldehyde resin is a condensation product of formaldehyde and *p*-tertiary-butylphenol, derived from a reaction mixture of formaldehyde (HCHO) with *p*-tert-butylphenol (PTBP) under the basic condition HCHO>PTBP. PTBP-FR is compounded as a tackifier in polychloroprene rubber adhesives for industrial and household uses. The adhesives are suitable for adhesion of rubber and leather; therefore the adhesives are used in manufacturing of shoes, handbags, watch straps, hats, belts, and other leather and rubber products. *p*-Tertiary-butylphenol formaldehyde is used in automotive industries as a sealant. It is used in waterproof glues, hence often in construction, e.g., wooden panels, plywood insulation, furniture, rock wool and fiberglass, hardboards, high-quality paper, and glossy fabrics and fabric labels.

p-Tertiary-butylphenol formaldehyde is occasionally found in inks, paints, lip liner, athletic tape, and plastic-nail adhesive, disinfectants, deodorants, insecticides, film developers, dental bonding materials, and plastic prostheses.

In addition, almost all cobblers repair shoes with glues containing this allergen. When shoes get wet, the *p*-tertiary-butylphenol formaldehyde in these glues is dissolved and comes in contact with the skin. Also, it may cause chemically induced vitiligo.

Products to Avoid   Avoid waterproof glues for leather and rubber products. Avoid direct contact with glued wood and sawdust from fiberglass and hardboard. It may also be necessary to avoid duplicating paper and glued fabric materials.

Cross-reactivity   *p*-Tertiary-butylphenol formaldehyde cross-reacts with *p*-tert-butylcatechol (PTBC).

Alternatives   Cyanoacrylate glues and sealants such as Loctite Permatex, Sta-Lok are alternatives.

References
1. Geldof BA, Roesyanto ID, Van Joost TH (1989) Clinical aspects of para-tertiary-butyl-phenolformaldehyde resin (PTBP-FR) allergy. Contact Dermatitis 21:312–315
2. Massone L, Anonide A, Borghi S, Usiglio D (1996) Sensitization to para-tertiary-butylphenolformaldehyde resin. Int J Dermatol 35:177–180
3. Estlander T, Kostiainen M, Jolanki R, Kanerva L (1998) Active sensitization and occupational allergic contact dermatitis caused by para-tertiary-butylcatechol. Contact Dermatitis 38:96–100

Tosylamide/Formaldehyde Resin

Carola Lidén

Designations

INCI Name. Tosylamide/formaldehyde resin.
Synonyms. Toluenesulfonamide formaldehyde resin;
benzenesulfonamide; 4-methyl-polymer with
formaldehyde; Santolite MHP; Santolite MS.
CAS No. 25035-71-6.

Test Preparations

- 10% pet. (allergen-patch-tape)
- Test with nail varnish: Paint the nail varnish on
  the test patch. Dry completely before application
  onto the skin for testing.

Occurrence

Most traditional nail varnishes and many nail hardeners contain tosylamide/formaldehyde resin, which is
the main ingredient. It occurs in some lacquers such
as vinyl lacquers and nitrocellulose lacquers. Tosyl-
amide/formaldehyde resin is used as a film former.

Products to Avoid

Traditional nail varnishes and nail hardeners should
be avoided, as well as some lacquers.

Cross-reactivity

Some persons allergic to tosylamide/formaldehyde
resin may react also to formaldehyde.

Alternatives

Some nail varnishes and nail hardeners do not contain tosylamide/formaldehyde resin, so the ingredients on the package of the cosmetic product should
be checked. Products labeled "formaldehyde free"
may contain tosylamide/formaldehyde resin.

References

1. De Groot AC, White IR (2001) Cosmetics and skin care products. In: Rycroft RJG, Menné T, Frosch PJ, Lepoittevin J-P (eds) Textbook of contact dermatitis, 3rd edn, chap 32. Springer, Berlin Heidelberg New York, pp 671–672
2. Lidén C, Berg M, Färm G, Wrangsjö K (1993) Nail varnish allergy with far-reaching consequences. Br J Dermatol 128:57–62